BOOK

OF

MEDICARE

Commentary to Help People
Understand Medicare Terminology

CARTER GRAY

CONTENTS

LIMIT OF LIABILITY/DISCLAIMER OF WARRANTY

While the author has used best efforts in preparing this book, it makes no representations or warranties with respect to the accuracy or completeness of the contents of this book and specifically disclaims any implied warranties of merchantability or fitness for a particular purpose. No warranty may be created or extended by sales representatives or written sales materials. The advice and strategies contained in herein may not be suitable for your situation. You should consult with a professional where appropriate. The author shall not be liable for any loss of profit or any other commercial damages, including but not limited to special, incidental, consequential, or other damages.

A nongovernment entity powered by Pacific Insurance Group, a health insurance agency. Extra benefits require enrollment in an MA plan and depend on whether you are eligible to enroll in an MA plan in your area. Benefits are available only in select areas. Pacific Insurance Group represents Medicare Advantage (HMO, PPO, PFFS, and PDP) organizations that have a Medicare contract. Enrollment depends on the plan's contract renewal. We do not offer every plan available in your area. Any information we provide is limited to our plans in your area. Please contact Medicare. gov or 1-800-MEDICARE to get information on all of your options.

Pacific Insurance Group offers a diverse range of plans across multiple markets, representing providers such as Accendo Insurance Company,

Aetna Better Health of Washington Inc, Aetna Health Inc, Aetna Life Insurance Company, Amerigroup Washington, Inc, Arcadian Health Plan Inc, Cigna Health and Life Insurance Company, Continental Life Insurance Company of Brentwood Tennessee, Health Net Life Insurance Company, Homesite Insurance Company of the Midwest, Humana Insurance Company, Humana Medical Plan of Utah Inc, Kaiser Foundation Health Plan of the Northwest, Mass Mutual Ascent Life Insurance Company, Molina Healthcare of Washington, Pacific Source Community Health Plans, Premera Blue Cross, Regence BlueShield, SilverScript Insurance Company, United Healthcare Benefits of Texas Inc, United Healthcare Insurance Company, Wellcare Health Insurance Company of Washington Inc, Wellcare of Washington Inc, and Wellcare Prescription Insurance Inc.

ACKNOWLEDGEMENTS

Book of Medicare would not have been possible without the amazing team at Pacific Insurance Group.

INTRODUCTION

Original Medicare was established in 1965 and covers services that are reasonable or necessary to save lives, improve health, and provide comfort before dying. Medicare is a government-funded healthcare program for people over the age of sixty-five and other eligible individuals. It is a complex system because it is made up of several different parts, each of which covers specific types of medical services. Additionally, the program is subject to changes and updates made by the government and insurance companies, which can make it difficult for individuals to stay informed about the latest rules, regulations, and product changes. Furthermore, Medicare is designed to work with private health insurance, so it can be difficult for people to understand how the two interact. This complexity is also due to its strict regulation and compliance with the Federal laws. While the full retirement age for Social Security has risen, Medicare eligibility is still generally age sixty-five, so more people will start to be eligible for Medicare before they begin taking an income stream from Social Security. There are roughly sixty-five million Medicare beneficiaries with around 10,000 becoming newly eligible every day. Furthermore, Medicare Part B premiums vary based on people's income level. Someone enrolled in Medicare Part B with a higher adjusted gross income will pay a surcharge on their Medicare Part B and Part D premiums which is typically something they do not know until they enroll. The surcharge for Part B can result in an Income-Related Monthly Adjusted Amount (IRMAA) ranging from a little to a lot. Eligible beneficiaries (people enrolled into Original

Medicare) with low incomes can receive assistance and pay nothing for their Medicare Part B premium. In addition to paying zero premium, some special needs plans give these beneficiaries monthly credit for groceries & utilities. These enhanced benefits for lower income individuals and extra surcharges to higher income individuals can lead to confusion.

Prescription drug benefits for people enrolled in Medicare can be overwhelming and confusing. Prescription Drug plans (also known as PDP's) change every year, so it is generally a good idea to compare multiple plans and speak with a local certified insurance agent to make sure the plan is suitable for the beneficiary. These agents should have the ability to compare plans to find the best overall solution, typically costing less money, enhancing benefits, or both. The prescriptions people take, and *how* they are filled (certain pharmacies or through the mail), can change the equation big time. If someone wants to pay as little as possible for their prescription drug costs, they should speak to an expert, be flexible, and open to making changes.

It is important for individuals to educate themselves about their options before making a decision about which Medicare plan to select because each plan can vary significantly in terms of coverage, cost, and out-of-pocket expenses. One should not get caught up in the letter or name of a plan, they should understand the cost and benefits in order to make the right decision. For example, some plans may have lower monthly premiums but higher out-of-pocket costs for medical services, while others may have higher monthly premiums but lower out-of-pocket costs. Additionally, each plan may cover different types of medical services, so it is important for individuals to understand their own healthcare needs and select a plan that will best meet those needs. Furthermore, the availability of a plan may vary depending on the location, so the options may be different for someone living in one area vs. another. Not being informed can lead to unexpected cost and coverage issues. Therefore, it is important to do research and consult with a local certified insurance agent to make the right informed decision.

The commentary in this book is intended to educate people on relevant facts around Medicare for people who want to discover the best route for their healthcare journey. Medigap/Medicare Supplement and Medicare Advantage Plans are NOT a "one size fits all" solution. Meaning, if someone says, "A Medicare Supplement Plan G is the best for everyone," or "A Medicare Advantage Prescription Drug plan is the only way to go," they are UNINFORMED. What works great for some people might be completely irrelevant for other beneficiaries. A lot of people have made bad decisions because of their unwillingness to stay informed with annual Medicare changes. Insurance agents in the Medicare arena are generally up to date because the Centers for Medicare & Medicaid Services (CMS) requires them to recertify each year in order to keep assisting beneficiaries with new plans. In addition, plan providers (typically insurance companies) require product training as well and have very high levels of compliance. It is recommended to sit down with a local certified insurance agent and calculate the right track forward.

HOW TO SIGN-UP FOR
ORIGINAL MEDICARE

Original Medicare is a fee-for-service healthcare program administered by the federal government. It consists of two parts: Medicare Part A (hospital insurance) and Medicare Part B (medical insurance). If someone is eligible for Original Medicare, they can sign up through the Social Security website **www.ssa.gov** or call Social Security at **1-800-772-1213**, or by visiting a local Social Security office. It is recommended to enroll in Original Medicare when first eligible to avoid paying late enrollment penalties and to have access to its healthcare coverage (unless someone has creditable coverage some other way).

Eligible beneficiaries can sign up for Original Medicare:

1. During the Initial Enrollment Period: Seven-month period, beginning three months before the beneficiary turns sixty-five years, the month they turn sixty-five years old, and three months after they turn sixty-five years. If an eligible beneficiary is already sixty-five years or older and not receiving Social Security or Railroad Retirement Board (RRB) benefits, they will most likely want to look at their options for enrolling in Medicare, unless they meet the criteria of still working and have creditable coverage.

2. During the General Enrollment Period: This is the period from January 1 to March 31 of each year. If an eligible beneficiary did not sign up for Medicare Part A and/or Part B during their Initial Enrollment Period, they can sign up during the General Enrollment Period. However, they may have to pay an ongoing late enrollment penalty if they did not sign up when first eligible.

3. If someone under age sixty-five has been receiving Social Security Disability Insurance (SSDI) or Railroad Retirement Board (RRB) benefits for at least twenty-four months, they will automatically be enrolled in Medicare Part A and Part B. They will receive a Medicare card in the mail around three months before their twenty-fifth month of disability benefits.

4. If someone has end-stage renal disease (ESRD) and they are in need of dialysis or a kidney transplant, they are eligible for Medicare, regardless of age.

Once a beneficiary has enrolled in Original Medicare, they will receive a red, white, and blue Medicare card which lists the beneficiaries' name and dates coverage became effective. It will also display their Medicare number, which serves as an identification number in the Medicare system. It is important to keep this card at all times and show it to healthcare providers when necessary.

WHY SIGN UP FOR
MEDIGAP
OR
A MAPD PLAN?

There are several reasons why someone who is eligible for Medicare may want to consider signing up for a Medigap or a Medicare Advantage Prescription Drug (MAPD) plan:

1. Original Medicare (Medicare Part A and Part B) does not cover all medical costs. There are deductibles, copayments, and coinsurance amounts a beneficiary will be responsible for paying out of their pocket. Medigap and MAPD plans can help cover these costs and make budgeting for healthcare expenses easier.

2. MAPD plans may also offer additional benefits, such as coverage for *prescription drugs, dental, vision*, and *hearing services* while providing a maximum out of pocket ceiling per calendar year.

3. Medigap and MAPD plans can offer more flexibility in choosing providers. With Original Medicare, a beneficiary may be limited to certain providers or have to pay more money to see a provider who is out of the Medicare network. With a Medigap or MAPD

plan, a beneficiary may have more flexibility in choosing providers, which can be especially important if they have a particular doctor or hospital they prefer.

4. Medigap/Medicare supplement plans are standardized private plans with a monthly fee that help cover some of the remaining costs like deductibles, coinsurance, and copays. Some plans offer coverage for services for medical care when traveling outside the United States.

ORIGINAL MEDICARE
PART A

Original Medicare Part A, also known as hospital insurance, is a federally funded healthcare program which provides coverage for medically necessary services and supplies. If someone has worked in the United States for forty quarters (ten years), they have likely paid for their Medicare Part A through FICA taxes. To be eligible for Medicare Part A, the beneficiary must be sixty-five years or older, or they must meet one of the following criteria:

- They are under sixty-five and have received Social Security Disability Insurance (SSDI) benefits for at least twenty-four months.

- They have End Stage Renal Disease (ESRD) and need dialysis or a kidney transplant.

- They have Lou Gehrig's disease (also known as amyotrophic lateral sclerosis or ALS).

(If a beneficiary is not eligible for Medicare Part A based on the above criteria, they may still be able to purchase it if they meet certain other conditions. The beneficiary can contact the Social Security Administration (SSA) to find out more about their eligibility for Medicare Part A.)

- Original Medicare Part A provides coverage for medically necessary:

  · Inpatient hospital care

  · Skilled nursing facility care

  · Home healthcare services

  · Acute care

  · Rehabilitation care

  · Skilled long-term care

  · Hospice care

- Original Medicare Part A also provides healthcare coverage as long as the care is medically necessary, and the services are ordered by a doctor. It is important to keep in mind that Original Medicare Part A has a deductible, and it does not cover all healthcare expenses.

STORY ABOUT
ADAM & PART A
MEDICARE

Growing up in Seattle, Adam always loved the smell of the salty Puget Sound. He was an avid runner and enjoyed staying active. Right out of college, Adam went to work for The Boeing Company. It was tumultuous times in the late 1960s and early 1970s in Seattle, commonly known as the "Boeing Bust" that didn't affect Adam's bright future; his college degree was a perfect fit for the popular Boeing 747. When Adam started working, he noticed something called FICA taking money from his paycheck, so on the weekend, he went to his local library and read up on how FICA works. Adam learned if people in the United States work forty quarters, they will be entitled to Original Medicare Part A. After a distinguished career at Boeing, Adam retired with a pension, social security, and a house paid off in Mukilteo overlooking the Puget Sound. Adam's favorite activity was to wake up every morning and run down to Lighthouse Park and breathe in his favorite air.

Adam had always been in great health, probably due to the marathons he loved to run. When he was first eligible for Original Medicare Part A, Adam logged into his social security portal and enrolled. One day while out on his usual morning jog, Adam tripped and fell on the pavement, hit his head, and was knocked unconscious. A passerby saw Adam lying on the ground and called for an ambulance. Adam was rushed to the emergency department, where he was diagnosed with a concussion. The doctors at the hospital decided to admit Adam for observation to monitor his concussion. Adam stayed in the hospital for a week, receiving round-the-clock care from a team of doctors and nurses.

When it was time for Adam to be discharged, he was worried about how he would pay for his medical bills because he was on a fixed income and did not have private health insurance. However, he remembered that he was enrolled in Medicare Part A, which covers hospitalization. Adam's Medicare Part A coverage helped pay for his hospital stay, including the cost of his room and board, medical supplies, and medications. It covered most of the cost of the medical procedures he received while in the hospital. A few weeks later, Adam drove his Midnight Blue 61' 409 Chevy Impala to the post office to pick up his mail and noticed medical bills for his Part A deductible and coinsurance. Adam knew it was time to get more educated on healthcare options so he could have more peace of mind going forward. Adam googled "Best Medicare Insurance Agency Near Me" and scheduled an appointment to speak with a local certified insurance agent. Adam discovered he could have spent ZERO dollars for a plan and lowered his medical bills from his accident.

Over the next few years, Adam made the most of his retirement. He traveled to visit his children and grandchildren, took up gardening as a hobby, and even volunteered at the local hospital to give back to the community. As the years passed, Adam remained grateful for the coverage Original Medicare Part A provided, but now he had a plan in place so if he ever tripped again, it would cost him much less. Adam was grateful to have Medicare Part A and was thankful it was there to help him when he had to go to the hospital.

ORIGINAL MEDICARE
PART B

- Original Medicare Part B, also known as medical insurance, is a federally funded healthcare program which provides coverage for medically necessary services and supplies. It is one part of the Original Medicare program. If someone does not enroll in Medicare Part B when they are eligible, they will most likely face a lifetime penalty (unless they have creditable coverage some other way).

- Original Medicare Part B provides 80 percent coverage for a wide range of medically necessary services and supplies, including:

  - Primary care physician visits
  - Outpatient care
  - Preventive care services
  - Durable medical equipment
  - Mental healthcare
  - Laboratory tests
  - X-rays and other diagnostic tests

- Original Medicare Part B includes a "Welcome to Medicare" preventive visit (during the first twelve months of enrollment for Medicare Part B). It also covers physical therapy and occupational therapy, as long as the care is medically necessary, and the services are ordered by a doctor.

- Original Medicare Part B has a monthly premium which is typically deducted from Social Security benefits or paid directly to the Medicare program. It also has a deductible and coinsurance for some services, and it does not cover all healthcare expenses.

- Original Medicare Part B can have an Income Related Monthly Adjusted Amount (IRMAA) added to the monthly Part B premium. IRMAA is an additional premium some Medicare beneficiaries are required to pay. It is based on the beneficiary's income, as reported on their tax return from two years prior.

STORY ABOUT
BETHANY & PART B
MEDICARE

Growing up, Bethany loved riding in her dad's Gypsy Red '57 Chevy; she knew she had the best dad in the world but hated the smell of his Marlboro Reds. Through the smokey air, her dad would remind her, "You can do anything a boy can do." Bethany will always remember July 21st, 1969, the day she witnessed Neil Armstrong walking on the moon. Remembering what her dad always said, Bethany went on to get a degree in aerospace and got a job at NASA right out of college.

Bethany had always been healthy and active. When she was first eligible for Original Medicare, Bethany logged into her Social Security portal and enrolled. She enjoyed hiking, gardening, and spending time with her grandchildren. However, one day she started experiencing some unusual symptoms. She had a persistent cough, shortness of breath, and fatigue. Concerned about her health, Bethany made an appointment to see her primary care doctor. After conducting a physical examination and ordering some tests, the doctor diagnosed Bethany with chronic obstructive pulmonary disease (COPD). COPD is a chronic respiratory condition that makes it difficult to breathe. It is often caused by long-term exposure to lung irritants, such as tobacco smoke. Bethany was shocked by the diagnosis. She had never smoked and had always taken good care of her health. However, she knew that she needed to take action to manage her condition. Bethany's doctor prescribed a number of medications to help control her symptoms and prevent further deterioration of her lung function. They also recommended she attend a rehabilitation program to help her improve her endurance and reduce her risk of respiratory infections. Bethany was able to get the medical treatment and support she needed to manage her COPD. After a few months of treatment, Bethany was feeling much better. Bethany was worried about how she would pay for her medical treatments because she was on a fixed income and did not have private health insurance. However, she remembered she was enrolled in Medicare Part B, which covers a wide range of medical services and supplies. Bethany's Medicare Part B coverage helped pay for her rehabilitation program, and it also covered 80 percent of the cost of her doctor's visits and any diagnostic tests that were needed to monitor her condition.

A few weeks later, Bethany drove her Sunfire Yellow 67' Corvette Stingray Convertible to the post office to pick up her mail; she opened medical bills for her Part B deductible and coinsurance amounts. Bethany realized it was time to get more educated on healthcare options so she could have more peace of mind going forward. Bethany googled "Best Medicare Insurance Agency Near Me" and scheduled an appointment to speak with a local certified insurance agent. Bethany discovered she could have spent ZERO dollars for a plan and lowered her medical bills from her medical treatments. Medicare Part B was a vital resource for Bethany as she navigated her health journey. It provided her with the coverage she needed to get the medical treatment and support she required, and it helped her with primary care expenses, but now she had an additional plan in place to fill in the gaps Part B didn't cover.

MEDICARE PART C
(MEDICARE ADVANTAGE PLANS)

- Medicare Part C, also known as Medicare Advantage Plans, are Medicare health plans offered by private insurance companies. These plans typically combine the benefits of Medicare Part A (hospital insurance) and Part B (medical insurance) with prescription drug coverage, all in one plan, which is then an MAPD plan.

- Medicare Advantage Plans must cover all of the same benefits as Original Medicare but generally offer additional benefits such as *prescriptions*, *dental*, *vision*, and *hearing* coverage. These plans are an alternative to Original Medicare and are available to those who are enrolled in Medicare Part A and Part B.

- MAPD plans include prescription drug coverage, which is not included in Original Medicare. This means a beneficiary enrolled in an MAPD plan does not need to purchase a separate Medicare Part D PDP.

- Medicare Advantage Plans may have network restrictions, which means the beneficiary may have to see certain providers or go to certain facilities in order to receive coverage. Not all Medicare Advantage Plans are available in all areas.

- MAPD plans range in premiums from ZERO dollars per month to typically less than $99 per month. MAPD plans protect people from potential financial catastrophe due to medical expenses because they have built-in-true-out-of-pocket maximums.

"It is a complete head scratcher as to why someone who is already enrolled in Original Medicare and cannot afford a Medigap plan, wouldn't pay ZERO dollars and sign up for an MAPD plan, but it happens all the time."

"Hemi"

(74-year-old wise man)

STORY ABOUT
CANDACE & PART C MEDICARE ADVANTAGE PRESCRIPTION DRUG (MAPD) PLAN

Candace's first memory was in the summer of 1954 when Bellevue, Washington was awarded the "All American City Award," and the entire town was filled with pride. Over the years, Candance watched her town expand and change, but she will always remember those weekends in high school bowling at Belle Lanes.

Candace had always been in good health, probably from the dance classes she attended every Friday night. When she was first eligible for Original Medicare, Candace logged into her Social Security portal and enrolled. After doing some research, Candace decided to enroll in an MAPD plan because it provided all the same coverage as Original Medicare, plus additional benefits for things like prescription drugs, vision, hearing, and dental care. Candace's Medicare Advantage plan covered her primary care visits and also covered preventive care services, such as flu shots and screenings for cancer.

Candace enjoyed spending time with her friends, traveling, and volunteering at her local animal shelter. However, as she got older, Candace started to have some issues with her health. She was diagnosed with high blood pressure, and she started taking a generic medication she received through the mail. One day, Candace discovered a lump on her breast and scheduled an appointment with her primary care physician who then ordered a mammogram. The results came back with some abnormalities, and Candace was referred to an oncologist who performed more extensive testing which resulted in her having a biopsy. The technician and doctors were all kind and compassionate, and Candace felt nurtured. She had a few sleepless nights, but the results came back negative which was great news. Candace was relieved to know her Medicare Advantage Plan would cover the majority of the costs associated with her medical expenses. Candace was grateful for the peace of mind Medicare Part C provided. After a few weeks, Candace was finally feeling like herself again.

As she drove home in her Pearl White 61' VW Bus, Candace decided to follow all of her doctor's instructions which included a mammogram every six months for two years. She knew that she had to be proactive about her health if she wanted to continue living a long and healthy life. Thanks to her MAPD plan, Candace was able to get the medical treatment she needed to manage her health journey. She also finally scheduled the hearing appointment she had been putting off since most MAPD plans include dental, vision, and hearing benefits.

MEDICARE PART D
PRESCRIPTION DRUG
(PDP) PLAN

- Medicare Part D helps cover the cost of prescription drugs; it is offered by private insurance companies and designed to work alongside Original Medicare. It is an optional program, which means the Medicare beneficiary does not have to enroll in a plan if they do not want prescription drug coverage. However, by not signing up for a Medicare Part D PDP when first eligible, a beneficiary will likely face a lifetime penalty if/when they decide to sign up later on.

- Medicare Part D premiums are paid directly to the private insurance company. It has a deductible, copayments, and coinsurance for some drugs. The out-of-pocket costs to the beneficiary will depend on the Part D plan selected.

- Medicare Part D does not cover all prescription drugs, and it does not cover drugs that are NOT medically necessary. It also does NOT cover drugs used for cosmetic purposes or for the treatment of weight loss or weight gain.

- Plans change every year, so it is wise to seek out a local insurance agent to make sure the beneficiary is in a plan that is suitable for their needs.

- Most Medicare drug plans have a coverage gap (also called the "donut hole"). This means there's a temporary limit on what the drug plan will cover for drugs.

STORY ABOUT
DEBORAH & PART D PRESCRIPTION DRUG (PDP) PLAN

Growing up in Snohomish, Washington next to a train depot, Deborah's first word was "train." She was mesmerized by the noises they made. As a child, one of Deborah's favorite past times was to grab a Green River fountain drink from Rexall's and watch the trains run through town on the Great Northern Railway. After high school, Deborah married a conductor for the Burlington Northern Railway and they had two children.

Deborah had always been in good health and diligent about saving for her golden years. When she was first eligible for Original Medicare, Deborah logged into her Social Security portal and enrolled.

After doing some research, Deborah decided to enroll in a Medicare Part D PDP. Medicare Part D is a voluntary prescription drug benefit available to individuals who are enrolled in Medicare. It is designed to help individuals afford the cost of prescription medications, which can be a significant burden for many people on a fixed income. She knew as she aged, she might need to take medications and wanted to make sure she had coverage for the cost. As Deborah got older, she started to have some issues with her health and was diagnosed with high cholesterol, high blood pressure, and type 2 diabetes. Her primary care physician prescribed a number of medications to help control her conditions.

Deborah's Medicare Part D Plan covered the majority of her prescription medications. She was required to pay the Part D deductible, a monthly premium for her plan as well as a copay or coinsurance for each prescription she filled. However, the drug costs were much lower than what she would have paid if she had to pay for her medications out of her pocket. In addition to the financial benefits, Deborah appreciated the convenience of having her prescription medications delivered to her doorstep. She no longer had to worry about driving her 69' Cortez Silver Camaro ZL1 to the pharmacy or remembering to refill her prescriptions. Thanks to her Medicare Part D coverage, Deborah was able to get the medications she needed to manage her health conditions. She was able to stay healthy and active, and she appreciated the convenience and financial support that her plan provided.

Over the next few years, Deborah's condition significantly improved thanks to the combination of proper treatment and medications. As Deborah returned to her normal routine, she made sure to follow all of her doctor's instructions and take good care of herself. She knew that she had to be proactive about her health if she wanted to continue living a long and healthy life. Medicare Part D provided her with the coverage she needed to afford her prescription medications and made managing her health easier and more convenient.

MEDICARE PLAN F
(MEDICARE SUPPLEMENT/MEDIGAP)

- Medicare Supplement Plan F, also known as Medigap Plan F, is a type of insurance which helps cover the gaps not covered by Original Medicare. These costs include Part A and B deductibles, copayments, and coinsurance. Medigap plans are offered by private insurance companies and are designed to work alongside Original Medicare.

- Medicare Plan F is a federally regulated standardized plan, which means it must follow certain rules set by the federal government. All Medicare Plan F plans must offer the same benefits regardless of which insurance company sells it.

- Medicare Plan F is one of many Medigap plans available in most states. It is considered a comprehensive plan, as it covers all medically necessary out-of-pocket costs not covered by Original Medicare Part A (hospital insurance) and Part B (medical insurance). This includes the Part A deductible, the Part B deductible, and the Part B coinsurance.

- Medicare Plan F provides comprehensive coverage for Original Medicare, which means the beneficiary will not have to pay any out-of-pocket costs for covered services approved by Medicare.

This can be particularly beneficial for those with high medical expenses or who need frequent medical care.

- Medicare Plan F is no longer available to those who became eligible for Medicare on or after January 1, 2020. However, those who were already enrolled in Medicare Plan F before this date can continue to use the plan.

- Medicare Plan F does not cover certain benefits, such as custodial long-term care, vision, hearing, and dental care. It also does not cover prescription drugs, which are covered under a separate Medicare Part D Plan at an additional cost.

STORY ABOUT
FELIX & PLAN F
(MEDIGAP)

Felix grew up in Forks, Washington, and sunlight was a joy for most people in town. For Felix who was a legendary steelhead fisherman, a little rain didn't bother him. The saying "a fish of a thousand casts" didn't apply to Felix; he was a natural from age nine. On April 17th, 1961, everyone was talking about the "Bay of Pigs" Cuban missile crisis; the only "Bay" on Felix's mind was Callam Bay where he caught his first fifty-pound King Salmon.

Felix had always been in good health, probably from all the wild fish he ate. When he was first eligible for Original Medicare, Felix met with a local certified insurance agent and decided to enroll in a Medicare Plan F, which is a supplement to Original Medicare (Part A and Part B) and started paying a monthly premium. He enjoyed fishing, woodworking, and spending time with his grandchildren. One of his favorite pastimes was to drive his 71' Plymouth Hemi Barracuda Convertible, a.k.a. "The Black Mamba," through the Olympic National Park. Felix thought it was the best medication possible. However, as he got older, Felix started to have some issues with his health. He was diagnosed with high blood pressure and type 2 diabetes.

One day, Felix had a heart attack and was rushed to the hospital. Felix was admitted and received top-notch medical care, including a triple bi-pass surgery and spent several days recovering in the hospital. Felix was relieved to know his Medicare Plan F would cover all the costs Original Medicare did not, such as his deductible and coinsurance. As he recuperated, Felix was grateful for the peace of mind his Medicare Plan F provided. The nurses and doctors were all kind and compassionate, and Felix felt well taken care of. After a few weeks, as Felix returned home, he made sure to follow all of his doctor's instructions and take better care of himself. Felix knew he had to be proactive about his health if he wanted to continue living a long and healthy life.

Felix was able to get the medical treatment and support he needed to manage his chronic conditions. He started seeing his primary care physician bi-annually and going to the gym. He was able to stay healthy and active and appreciated the comprehensive coverage his Medicare Plan F provided. Overall, Medicare Plan F was a valuable resource for Felix as he navigated his healthcare journey, and he never received any medicals bills in the mail.

MEDICARE PLAN G
(MEDICARE SUPPLEMENT/MEDIGAP)

- Medicare Supplement Plan G, also known as Medigap Plan G, is a type of insurance that helps cover the gaps not covered by Original Medicare. These costs include the Part A deductible, copayments, and coinsurance. Medigap plans are offered by private insurance companies and are designed to work alongside Original Medicare.

- Medicare Plan G is a standardized plan that is federally regulated, which means it must follow certain rules set by the federal government. All Medicare Plan G policies must offer the same benefits regardless of which insurance company offers it.

- Medicare Plan G is one of many Medigap plans available in most states. It is considered a comprehensive plan, as it covers all of the out-of-pocket costs for Original Medicare Part A (hospital insurance) and Part B (medical insurance) except for the Part B deductible. This can be particularly beneficial for those with high medical expenses or who need frequent medical care.

- Medicare Plan G does not cover certain benefits, such as custodial long-term care, vision, hearing, and dental care. It also does not cover prescription drugs, which are covered under the separate Medicare Part D program at an additional cost.

STORY ABOUT
GABRIEL & PLAN G
(MEDIGAP)

Growing up in rural eastern Washington, Gabriel learned the importance of irrigation, which can turn a desert into farmland. Gabriel loved watching crops go from seed to harvest. In 1980, Mount St. Helens erupted and covered the majority of eastern Washington with ash because the winds were blowing to the east. At first, it looked like the mother of all thunderstorms, but when the ash started falling, it was like a dark blizzard, and it became eerily quiet. The next morning, the land was unrecognizable, the crops were likely going to die, and it took weeks to wash the ash off the buildings.

Gabriel's health got a little worse over the years, probably from his wife's delicious homemade cooking with a lot of salt and butter. When he was first eligible for Original Medicare, Gabriel met with a local certified insurance agent and decided to enroll in a Medicare Plan G, which is a supplement to Original Medicare (Part A and Part B) and started paying a monthly premium. Medicare Plan G is a comprehensive plan that covers a wide range of out-of-pocket costs. The main difference between Medicare Plan F and Plan G is that Plan G does not cover the Medicare Part B deductible.

One day, Gabriel had a stroke and was rushed to the hospital. He was admitted and received inpatient care followed by rehabilitation care which took several days to recover in the hospital. Gabriel was relieved to know that his Medicare Plan G would cover the cost of his Original Medicare deductible and coinsurance. As he recuperated, Gabriel was grateful for Original Medicare along with his Medicare Plan G, and he knew that he didn't have to worry about how he was going to pay for his medical bills and could focus on getting better.

After a few weeks, Gabriel was feeling like himself again, especially once he got back into his Skyline Blue 64' Pontiac GTO when his wife was finally able to drive him home. Gabriel made sure to follow all of his doctor's instructions and take good care of himself, which meant only one slice of his wife's famous apple pie on Sundays. He knew that he had to be proactive about his health if he wanted to continue living a long and healthy life. Gabriel started seeing his primary care physician bi-annually and patiently tolerated every MRI his doctor felt was medically necessary.

Over the next few years, Gabriel made the most of his retirement; he took up painting as a hobby, traveled to visit his children and grandchildren, and even volunteered at the local library to give back to the community. Thanks to his Medicare Plan G coverage, Gabriel was able to get the medical treatment and support he needed to manage his condition. He was able to stay healthy and active, and he appreciated the financial support that his plan provided. In addition to the medical benefits, Gabriel appreciated the convenience of having his out-of-pocket costs covered by his Medicare Plan G.

MEDICARE PLAN N
(MEDICARE SUPPLEMENT/MEDIGAP)

- Medicare Supplement Plan N, also known as Medigap Plan N, is a type of insurance that helps cover the gaps not covered by Original Medicare. Medigap plans are offered by private insurance companies and are designed to work alongside Original Medicare.

- Medicare Plan N is a standardized plan that is federally regulated, which means it must follow certain rules set by the federal government. All Medicare Plan N policies must offer the same benefits, regardless of which insurance company offers it.

- Medicare Plan N is one of many Medigap plans available in most states. It is considered a mid-range option, with lower monthly premiums. Medicare Plan N does not cover certain benefits, including the Part B deductible. It has higher out-of-pocket costs than some of the other Medigap plans because of copayments for some services. For example, Medicare Plan N requires a copayment for office visits and emergency room visits that don't result in an inpatient admission.

- Medicare Plan N does not cover certain benefits, such as custodial long-term care, vision, hearing, and dental care. It also does not cover prescription drugs, which can be covered under a separate Medicare Part D Plan.

STORY ABOUT
NATHANIEL & PLAN N
(MEDIGAP)

Growing up, Nathaniel loved malts from the local drive-in restaurant, cruising around town, and going to the drive-in movie theater. One Friday night, Nathaniel got into his Candy Apple Red 66' Ford Mustang and took his girlfriend to see *The Russians Are Coming, the Russians Are Coming*. The movie peaked his interest in maritime activities when he was in high school, and that's how his career at the yacht club got started.

Nathaniel had always been in good health except for the brains cells he lost from being a hippie in his youth. When Nathaniel was first eligible for Original Medicare, he met with a local certified insurance agent and decided to enroll in a Medicare Plan N, which is a supplement to Original Medicare (Part A and Part B), and started paying a monthly premium. Medicare Plan N is a comprehensive plan that covers a wide range of out-of-pocket costs. The main difference between Medicare Plan N and the other Medigap plans is Plan N requires the beneficiary to pay a portion of the out-of-pocket costs associated with Original Medicare. Specifically, Plan N requires the beneficiary to pay copayments. Despite the additional out-of-pocket costs, Nathaniel appreciated the comprehensive coverage provided by his Medicare Plan N. It gave him the peace of mind of knowing that he was covered for a wide range of medical expenses, and it helped ease the financial burden of paying for his medical treatment.

One day, Nathaniel had a mental breakdown, and his friend took him to the emergency room. The hospital did not admit Nathaniel because he started to feel better a few hours later, and it only cost him a small copayment because his Medicare Plan N covered the rest of the bill. The next day Nathaniel scheduled an appointment to see a clinical psychologist, and after a few months of treatment and medication, Nathaniel started to feel normal again. Nathaniel was grateful for his Medicare Plan N and knew he didn't have to worry about how he was going to pay for his medical bills.

As Nathaniel returned home, he made sure to follow all of his doctor's instructions which included screenings for depression and "talk therapy." Nathaniel knew he had to be proactive about his health if he wanted to continue living a long and healthy life. Over the next few years, Nathaniel made the most of his retirement. He took up gardening as a hobby, traveled to visit his children and grandchildren, and cruised around in his 66' Mustang. Overall, Medicare Plan N was a valuable resource for Nathaniel as he navigated his health journey. It provided him with the coverage he needed to afford his medical treatment and made managing his health easier and more convenient.

TYPES OF
MEDICARE
ADVANTAGE PLANS

- MAPD (Medicare Advantage Prescription Drug Plan)
- HMO (Health Maintenance Organization)
- HMO POS (HMO Point of Service)
- PPO (Preferred Provider Organization)
- LPPO (Local Preferred Provider Organization)
- PFFS (Private Fee-for-Service)
- MSA (Medicare Savings Account)
- MCP (Medicare Cost Plan)
- PACE (Programs of All-Inclusive Care for The Elderly)
- MMP (Medicare Advantage Medicare-Medicaid Plan)
- HMO-SNP (Special Needs Plan)

Medicare Advantage Prescription Drug (MAPD) Plans are types of Medicare Advantage Plans that include prescription drug coverage. They provide an alternative to traditional Medicare and a standalone PDP (Part D). MAPDs are required to provide all the same benefits as Original Medicare, including hospital care, doctor services, and preventive care. They also include coverage for prescription drugs, which is provided through the private insurance company. The benefit design, costs, and the formulary of drugs covered may vary among the different plans. MAPDs are available in certain areas and are limited to Medicare beneficiaries who are enrolled in a Medicare Advantage plan. Some Medicare Advantage plans (such as HMOs and PPOs) include prescription drug coverage as part of their plan, while other plans may require enrolling in a separate PDP (Part D) to have drug coverage. An MAPD Plan may be a good option for Medicare beneficiaries who require regular medication and want to have their medical and prescription drug coverage in one plan. Some of the following factors may indicate that an MAPD plan is a good fit for someone:

- They are currently enrolled in a Medicare Advantage plan without prescription drug coverage, and they need regular medications.

- They want to have their medical and prescription drug coverage in one plan.

- They want to have predictable out-of-pocket costs.

- They have a chronic condition that requires regular medication.

- They have a limited budget and want to avoid high out-of-pocket costs for prescription drugs.

- They prefer to have a predictable formulary of drugs covered by the plan.

Medicare Advantage Health Maintenance Organizations (HMOs) are a type of Medicare Advantage Plan offered by private insurance companies. These plans provide an alternative to traditional Medicare and typically offer lower out-of-pocket costs than original Medicare. HMOs are designed to provide comprehensive health coverage through a network of providers. Typically, members must choose a primary care physician who acts as a gatekeeper and must be seen by this physician before they can see any other providers. This primary care physician is responsible for coordinating all of the member's healthcare needs and making referrals to specialists as needed. Benefits covered under a Medicare Advantage HMO plan include hospital care, doctor services, preventive care, and prescription drug coverage. The benefits and cost-sharing for these plans can vary depending on the plan and the location. HMOs typically have more restrictive provider networks than other types of Medicare Advantage Plans, like Preferred Provider Organizations (PPOs) and Private Fee-for-Service (PFFS) plans. This means members must receive care from providers within the HMO's network, with few exceptions. Additionally, members of a Medicare Advantage HMO plan must live within the service area of the plan they enroll in. It's important to note that while Medicare Advantage HMOs can offer lower out-of-pocket costs, they also have more restrictive networks and require referrals from primary care physicians to see specialists.

Medicare Advantage Health Maintenance Organization Point of Service Plans (HMO POS) are types of Medicare Advantage Plans offered by private insurance companies. These plans are similar to traditional HMOs, but they provide more flexibility in terms of accessing out-of-network providers. Like traditional HMOs, HMO POS plans require members to select a primary care physician who acts as a gatekeeper, coordinating the member's healthcare needs and making referrals to specialists as needed. However, HMO POS plans also allow members to see out-of-network providers, typically with a referral from the primary care physician and with higher out-of-pocket costs. Benefits covered under a Medicare Advantage HMO POS plan include hospital care, doctor services, preventive care, and prescription drug coverage. The benefits and cost-sharing for these plans can vary depending on the plan and the location. It's important to note that while HMO POS plans offer more flexibility in accessing out-of-network providers, they also have higher out-of-pocket costs for those services.

Medicare Advantage Preferred Provider Organizations (PPOs) are types of Medicare Advantage Plans offered by private insurance companies. They provide an alternative to traditional Medicare and generally offer more flexibility in terms of accessing providers than other types of Medicare Advantage Plans such as HMOs or POS plans. In a Medicare Advantage PPO plan, members are typically not required to choose a primary care physician or obtain referrals to see specialists. Instead, they can see any provider within the plan's network without a referral, although they may pay more if they see a provider outside of the network. Benefits covered under a Medicare Advantage PPO plan include hospital care, doctor services, preventive care, and prescription drug coverage. The benefits and cost-sharing for these plans can vary depending on the plan and the location. PPOs typically have a wider provider network than HMOs, which can make it easier for members to access care and see the providers they prefer. However, it's important to note that while PPOs offer more flexibility in accessing providers, they may also have higher out-of-pocket costs than other types of Medicare Advantage Plans.

Local Preferred Provider Organizations (LPPOs) are types of Medicare Advantage Plans offered by private insurance companies contracted with a specific network of healthcare providers. This means that the plan's members generally have lower out-of-pocket costs if they receive care from providers within the plan's network. These plans typically include additional benefits, such as vision, hearing, and dental coverage, which are not covered under original Medicare.

Medicare Advantage Private Fee-for-Service (PFFS) plans are types of Medicare Advantage Plans offered by private insurance companies. These plans provide an alternative to traditional Medicare and offer more flexibility in terms of accessing providers than other types of Medicare Advantage Plans such as HMOs or PPOs. In a Medicare Advantage PFFS plan, members are typically not required to choose a primary care physician or obtain referrals to see specialists. Instead, they can see any provider that accepts the plan's terms and conditions, regardless of whether the provider is part of the plan's network. Benefits covered under a Medicare Advantage PFFS plan include hospital care, doctor services, preventive care, and prescription drug coverage. The benefits and cost-sharing for these plans can vary depending on the plan and the location. PFFS plans typically have no network restrictions, and the members can see any provider that accepts the plan's terms and conditions. However, it's important to note that while PFFS plans offer more flexibility in accessing providers, they also may have higher out-of-pocket costs than other types of Medicare Advantage Plans.

Medicare Advantage Medicare Savings Account (MSA) are types of Medicare Advantage Plans offered by private insurance companies. These plans are designed to provide an alternative to traditional Medicare and are only available to individuals who meet certain income and asset requirements. MSA plans combine a high-deductible Medicare Advantage Plan with a savings account that is used to pay for healthcare expenses. Members are required to pay for their healthcare expenses up to the plan's deductible, and then the plan pays for covered expenses. Any money left in the savings account at the end of the year can be rolled over to the next year or withdrawn by the member. Benefits covered under a Medicare Advantage MSA plan include hospital care, doctor services, preventive care, and prescription drug coverage. The benefits and cost-sharing for these plans can vary depending on the plan and the location. It's important to note that MSA plans are only available to a limited number of beneficiaries, usually those with lower incomes, and availability varies by location. Additionally, the member is responsible for managing the savings account and the funds in it and making sure to have enough money in the account to cover their healthcare expenses.

Medicare Advantage Cost Plans (MCP) are types of Medicare Advantage Plans offered by private insurance companies. These plans provide an alternative to traditional Medicare and typically cover the same benefits as Original Medicare, including hospital care, doctor services, preventive care, and prescription drug coverage. Medicare Advantage Cost Plans are different from other Medicare Advantage Plans because they are not required to offer a network of providers, meaning members can see any provider that accepts Medicare. They also cover out-of-network services, but members may pay higher out-of-pocket costs for those services. Cost plans are typically offered in certain areas where there are few Medicare Advantage options available. They can be a good choice for people who want to keep the same doctors and hospitals, or who want to have the flexibility to see any provider who accepts Medicare. It's important to note that while Cost plans offer more flexibility in accessing providers, they also may have higher out-of-pocket costs than other types of Medicare Advantage Plans. Additionally, they may not be offered in all areas and availability may vary.

Medicare Advantage Program of All-Inclusive Care for the Elderly (PACE) are types of Medicare Advantage Plans offered by private insurance companies. These plans provide an alternative to traditional Medicare and are designed to meet the unique healthcare needs of older adults with chronic care needs. PACE plans provide comprehensive and coordinated care to older adults who are at risk of nursing home placement. They offer a range of services, including primary care, hospital care, prescription drugs, home healthcare, and long-term care services. They also provide social and recreational services to help older adults maintain their independence and quality of life. PACE plans are required to provide all the same benefits as Original Medicare, including hospital care, doctor services, preventive care, and prescription drug coverage. They also provide additional benefits such as transportation and meals, as well as social and recreational services. PACE plans are only available in certain areas and are limited to Medicare beneficiaries who are fifty-five years of age or older and who meet certain functional and financial eligibility criteria. It's important for a beneficiary to evaluate their specific healthcare needs and preferences before deciding if a PACE plan is the right fit for them. It's recommended to compare the available options and costs, as well as the level of coverage and the providers available in the plan's network, to determine if this type of plan is the right fit for them.

Medicare Advantage Medicare-Medicaid Plan (MMP) are types of Medicare Advantage Plans offered by private insurance companies. These plans provide an alternative to traditional Medicare and Medicaid and are designed to meet the unique healthcare needs of certain Medicare beneficiaries, such as those who are dually eligible for Medicare and Medicaid. MMPs are required to provide all the same benefits as Original Medicare and Medicaid, including hospital care, doctor services, preventive care, prescription drug coverage, and long-term care services. They also provide additional benefits and services that are tailored to the specific needs of the population they serve. These benefits may include additional coverage for transportation to and from medical appointments, case management, and disease management programs. MMPs are available in certain states, and availability varies by location. Eligibility for these plans is determined by the state and the plan, typically based on income, specific assets, and Medicaid eligibility. It's important to note that not all Medicare beneficiaries are eligible for MMPs, and availability varies by location.

Medicare Advantage Special Needs Plans (SNPs) are types of Medicare Advantage Plans offered by private insurance companies. These plans are specifically designed to meet the unique healthcare needs of certain Medicare beneficiaries, such as those with chronic conditions, those who live in certain types of institutions, or those who are dually eligible. SNPs typically have more restrictive provider networks than other types of Medicare Advantage Plans, and they are required to provide additional benefits and services that are tailored to the specific needs of the population they serve. For example, an SNP for individuals with chronic conditions may offer additional benefits such as disease management programs or transportation to and from medical appointments. It's important to note, not all Medicare beneficiaries are eligible for SNPs and availability varies by location. SNPs are required to provide all the same benefits as other Medicare Advantage plans, including hospital care, doctor services, preventive care, and prescription drug coverage. Some examples of the beneficiaries that can be eligible for SNP plans are:

- Individuals with chronic conditions such as diabetes, heart failure, and ESRD
- People who live in skilled nursing facilities
- People who are dually eligible for both Medicare and Medicaid

GLOSSARY

* If the beneficiary has any questions about any of the following terms, it is recommended to contact the plan directly or speak with a Medicare representative. The beneficiary should discuss options with a healthcare provider to consider factors such as cost, convenience, and the specific needs of any medical condition.

A

Accountable Care Organizations (ACO): Groups of doctors, hospitals, and other healthcare professionals working together to give high-quality, coordinated service and healthcare.

- An ACO is a healthcare delivery model that aims to coordinate and improve the quality of care for a specific patient population while also reducing costs. ACOs bring together hospitals, doctors, and other healthcare providers to work as a team to provide coordinated, high-quality care to their patients.

- ACOs were first introduced by the Affordable Care Act (ACA) in 2010 as a way to encourage healthcare providers to work together and be more accountable for the overall health of their patients. ACOs are meant to be an alternative to the traditional fee-for-service model, where healthcare providers are paid for each service they provide, regardless of the overall health outcomes of their patients.

- Under the ACO model, healthcare providers are held accountable for the quality and cost of care they provide. They are given financial incentives to keep their patients healthy and prevent costly hospitalizations or other unnecessary medical procedures. ACOs are also responsible for tracking the health of their patients and using data to identify and address any potential issues before they become more serious and costly to treat.

- There are several different types of ACOs, including Medicare ACOs, Medicaid ACOs, and commercial ACOs. Medicare ACOs are designed to serve the needs of Medicare beneficiaries, while Medicaid ACOs serve Medicaid beneficiaries. Commercial ACOs serve patients with private insurance.

- ACOs can be structured in different ways, including as a network of independent healthcare providers or as a single entity. ACOs may also be structured as a for-profit or non-profit organization.

- There are several benefits to the ACO model. By coordinating care and working together as a team, ACOs can improve the quality of care for their patients and reduce costs by preventing unnecessary hospitalizations and other costly medical procedures. ACOs also provide patients with a single point of contact for their healthcare needs, which can make it easier for them to navigate the healthcare system.

- Overall, ACOs are an innovative healthcare delivery model that aims to coordinate and improve the quality of care for a specific patient population, while also reducing costs. While there are challenges to the ACO model, it has the potential to greatly improve the healthcare system and the overall health of patients.

Advance Beneficiary Notice of Noncoverage (ABN): In Original Medicare, a notice that a doctor, supplier, or provider gives a person with Medicare before furnishing an item or service if the doctor, supplier, or provider believes that Medicare may deny payment. In this situation, if the beneficiary isn't given an ABN before the item or service is provided, and Medicare denies payment, then the beneficiary may not have to pay for it. If the beneficiary is given an ABN, and signs it, the beneficiary may have to pay for the item or service if Medicare denies payment.

- The ABN is a form used by healthcare providers to inform Medicare beneficiaries they may be responsible for paying for a particular service or item that is not covered by Medicare. The ABN is not a guarantee that Medicare will not pay for the service or item, but it serves as a way to alert beneficiaries that they may be responsible for paying for it out-of-pocket.

- The ABN is required by Medicare in certain circumstances, such as when a service or item is considered experimental or investigational, or when it is not medically necessary. In these cases, the ABN is used to inform the beneficiary they may be responsible for paying for the service or item.

- The ABN is also used when a service or item may be covered by Medicare, but the provider is unsure if it will be covered in the specific case. In this situation, the ABN is used to inform the beneficiary that they may be responsible for paying for the service or item if it is not covered by Medicare.

- There are two types of ABNs: the Standard Form ABN and the Customized Form ABN. The Standard Form ABN is used in most situations and is provided by Medicare. The Customized Form ABN is used in rare circumstances and is developed by the provider.

- The ABN is an important tool for healthcare providers to use in situations where Medicare coverage may not be available. It allows beneficiaries to make informed decisions about their healthcare and to be prepared for any potential out-of-pocket expenses. It is important for beneficiaries to carefully read and understand the ABN and to ask any questions they may have before receiving a service or item that may not be covered by Medicare.

Advance Coverage Decision (ACD): A notice a beneficiary receives from a Medicare Advantage Plan letting them know in advance whether it will cover a particular service.

- Medicare's ACD process allows beneficiaries to request a determination on whether a specific service, item, or treatment will be covered by Medicare before it is received. The ACD process is meant to help beneficiaries make informed decisions about their healthcare and to avoid unexpected out-of-pocket expenses.

- The ACD process is available for all Medicare beneficiaries, but it is especially useful for those who are considering a new treatment or procedure that may not be covered by Medicare. It is also useful for those who are unsure if a service or item is covered by Medicare or if it is considered medically necessary.

- To request an ACD, beneficiaries must complete a Medicare Advance Coverage Determination Request form and submit it to their Medicare Administrative Contractor (MAC). The MAC will review the request and decide on whether the service, item, or treatment will be covered by Medicare.

- The ACD process is not meant to be a substitute for seeking medical advice from a healthcare provider. It is only meant to provide information on whether a service, item, or treatment will be covered by Medicare. Beneficiaries should always discuss their healthcare needs with their healthcare provider before making any decisions about their treatment.

- The ACD process can be a useful tool for beneficiaries who are considering a new treatment or procedure and want to know if it will be covered by Medicare. It can help them make informed decisions about their healthcare and avoid unexpected out-of-pocket expenses.

Advance Directive: A written document stating how an individual wants medical decisions to be made if the ability to make such decisions is lost. It may include a living will and a durable power of attorney for healthcare.

- Advance Directive is a document which allows individuals to specify their healthcare preferences and decisions in advance, in the event that they are unable to make their own decisions due to a serious illness or injury. The Advance Directive is also known as a living will or healthcare power of attorney.

- There are two main types of Advance Directives: the living will and the healthcare power of attorney. The living will allows individuals to specify their preferences for medical treatment in the event they are unable to make their own decisions. The healthcare power of attorney, also known as a durable power of attorney for healthcare, allows individuals to appoint someone else to make healthcare decisions on their behalf if they are unable to do so.

- It is important for individuals to consider creating a Medicare Advance Directive as part of their overall healthcare planning. A Medicare Advance Directive can help ensure that an individual's healthcare wishes are followed if they are unable to communicate them. It can also help alleviate the burden on family members or loved ones who may be asked to make decisions on the individual's behalf.

- Individuals can create an Advance Directive at any age, and it is a good idea to review and update the document periodically to ensure that it reflects their current wishes and preferences. It is also important to discuss the Advance Directive with family members, loved ones, and healthcare providers to ensure everyone is aware of the individual's preferences and decisions.

- Creating an Advance Directive is a personal decision that each individual should make based on their own circumstances and preferences. It is an important part of overall healthcare planning and can help ensure that an individual's wishes are followed if they are unable to make their own decisions due to a serious illness or injury.

ALS: Amyotrophic lateral sclerosis, also known as Lou Gehrig's disease.

- ALS, also known as Lou Gehrig's disease, is a progressive and ultimately fatal neurological disorder that affects nerve cells in the brain and spinal cord. The disease is characterized by the degeneration of motor neurons, which are responsible for transmitting signals from the brain to the muscles throughout the body. As the motor neurons die, the brain loses its ability to control muscle movement, leading to muscle weakness, atrophy, and, ultimately, paralysis.

- There is no cure for ALS, and treatment options are limited. The primary goal of treatment is to slow the progression of the disease and to manage symptoms. This may include medications to reduce muscle spasms, physical therapy to maintain muscle strength and mobility, and respiratory therapy to help with breathing difficulties.

- If a beneficiary or their loved one has been diagnosed with ALS, it is important to know Medicare covers many of the treatments and services related to the disease. This includes medications, durable medical equipment (DME) (such as wheelchairs and ventilators), and medical visits. In addition, Medicare may cover certain inpatient and outpatient rehabilitation services, as well as home healthcare services for those with severe mobility limitations.

- It is important to note that coverage for certain treatments and services may vary depending on the specific Medicare plan a beneficiary has. For example, some plans may have limits on the number of physical therapy sessions covered or may require the beneficiary to pay a copayment or deductible for certain services. It is also important to be aware that Medicare does not cover experimental or investigational treatments for ALS.

Ambulatory Surgical Center (ASC): A facility where certain surgeries may be performed for patients who aren't expected to need more than twenty-four hours of care.

- An ASC is a medical facility which specializes in providing same-day surgical care. This means patients who undergo procedures at an ASC are typically able to go home on the same day, rather than being required to stay overnight in a hospital. ASCs are typically focused on providing a limited range of surgical procedures that do not require an overnight stay.

- It is important to note that Medicare coverage for ASC services may vary depending on the specific Medicare plan a beneficiary has. Some plans may require a copayment or a deductible for certain services or may have limits on the number of covered procedures. It is also important to be aware that Medicare does not cover all procedures performed at an ASC. For example,

Medicare does not cover cosmetic surgery or procedures that are considered experimental or investigational.

Annual Election Period: Also known as the AEP. This runs from October 15th through December 7th. During this time Medicare Advantage and Medicare Part D plans can be changed with no restrictions.

- The Medicare Annual Election Period (AEP) is the time each year during which people who are enrolled in Medicare Advantage Plans or Medicare Part D PDPs can make changes to their coverage. It runs from October 15 to December 7, and during this time, beneficiaries can switch from one Medicare Advantage Plan to another, switch from a Medicare Advantage Plan back to Original Medicare, enroll in a Medicare Part D plan, or switch from one Medicare Part D plan to another.

- The Medicare AEP is important because it provides beneficiaries with an opportunity to review and make changes to their Medicare coverage if necessary. This allows beneficiaries to ensure that their coverage meets their current healthcare needs and that they are taking advantage of the best available options for their particular circumstances. Additionally, during AEP, beneficiaries can compare costs, coverage, and other important factors when choosing or changing their Medicare coverage. Failing to make changes during the AEP could result in beneficiaries being stuck with coverage that is no longer suitable for their needs for an entire year, so it is an important period for beneficiaries to take advantage of.

Appeal: An appeal is the action a beneficiary can take if they disagree with a coverage or payment decision made by Medicare, by their Medicare health plan, or by their Medicare Prescription Drug Plan. An appeal can be made if Medicare or the beneficiary's plan denies one of these:

- A request for a healthcare service, supply, item, or prescription drug that the beneficiary believes they should be able to get.

- A request for payment for a healthcare service, supply, item, or prescription drug the beneficiary already got.

- A request to change the amount the beneficiary must pay for a healthcare service, supply, item, or prescription drug.

A beneficiary can also appeal if Medicare or their plan stops providing or paying for all or part of a service, supply, item, or prescription drug the beneficiary believes they still need.

- If a beneficiary is enrolled in Medicare and disagrees with a coverage or payment decision made by their Medicare plan, the beneficiary has the right to appeal that decision. The Medicare appeal process is a way for the beneficiary to have a case reviewed by a higher level of decision-making authority within their plan or by an independent organization.

- There are four levels of appeal within the Medicare system:

  - Reconsideration: If a beneficiary disagrees with the decision made at the redetermination level, they can request a reconsideration. This level of appeal is handled by an independent organization known as a Qualified Independent Contractor (QIC).

· Redetermination: This is the first level of appeal and is handled by a beneficiary's Medicare plan. If the beneficiary disagrees with a coverage or payment decision made by their plan, they can request a redetermination by filling out a Medicare claim appeal form and submitting it to their plan.

· Administrative Law Judge (ALJ) hearing: If a beneficiary disagrees with the decision made at the reconsideration level, they can request an ALJ hearing. This level of appeal is handled by an ALJ who is independent of the Medicare system.

· Medicare Appeals Council (MAC) review: If a beneficiary disagrees with the decision made at the ALJ hearing, they can request a review by the MAC. The MAC is a group of ALJs who review decisions made at the ALJ level.

• It is important to note that the Medicare appeal process can be complex and time-consuming, and it is recommended that the beneficiary seeks the assistance of a healthcare professional or advocate if they are considering appealing a coverage or payment decision. It is also important to be aware that there are deadlines for requesting each level of appeal, so it is important to act promptly if they wish to appeal a decision.

Assignment of Benefits: An agreement by a doctor, provider, or supplier to be paid directly by Medicare, to accept the payment amount Medicare approves for the service, and not to bill the beneficiary for any more than the Medicare deductible and coinsurance.

• Assignment is a term used to describe the agreement between a healthcare provider and Medicare to accept the

Medicare-approved amount as payment in full for covered services. When a provider agrees to accept assignment, they agree to bill Medicare directly for the services they provide to Medicare beneficiaries and to accept the Medicare-approved amount as payment in full.

- If a beneficiary is enrolled in Medicare, and they visit a provider who accepts assignment, they may be responsible for paying a copayment or coinsurance for certain services. These out-of-pocket costs are typically a small percentage of the overall cost of the service and are required to be paid at the time the service is provided.

- It is important to note that not all providers accept assignments. Some providers may choose to bill Medicare directly for the services they provide but may also bill the beneficiary for any amount not covered by Medicare. This is known as nonassigned billing, and it is important to be aware the beneficiary may be responsible for paying a larger out-of-pocket cost if they visit a provider who does not accept assignment.

- If a beneficiary is considering receiving medical care from a provider who does not accept assignment, it is recommended they discuss the costs of the services with the provider and confirm whether they will be responsible for paying any additional out-of-pocket costs.

B

Beneficiary and Family Centered Care–Quality Improvement Organization (BFCC-QIO): A type of a QIO (an organization under contract with Medicare) that uses doctors and other healthcare experts to review complaints and quality of care for people with Medicare. The BFCC-QIO makes sure there is consistency in the case review process

while taking into consideration local factors and needs, including general quality of care and medical necessity.

- The BFCC-QIO is an organization that works to improve the quality of healthcare for Medicare beneficiaries and their families. The BFCC-QIO is responsible for conducting reviews of the quality of care provided to Medicare beneficiaries, as well as providing education and assistance to beneficiaries and their families on issues related to healthcare quality and patient safety.

- One of the primary roles of the BFCC-QIO is to review and make decisions on appeals related to the quality of care received by Medicare beneficiaries. If someone is a Medicare beneficiary and they are dissatisfied with the quality of care they have received, they can contact the BFCC-QIO to request a review of their case. The BFCC-QIO will work with the beneficiary and their healthcare providers to identify any issues with the care they received and to determine the appropriate course of action.

- In addition to its role in reviewing appeals, the BFCC-QIO also works to improve the overall quality of care provided to Medicare beneficiaries. This may include conducting studies to identify trends and patterns in healthcare quality, developing educational materials and resources for beneficiaries and their families, and working with healthcare providers to implement best practices and improve patient safety.

- If a Medicare beneficiary has questions or concerns about the quality of care they have received, it is recommended that they contact the BFCC-QIO for assistance. The beneficiary can find contact information for the BFCC-QIO in their state on the Medicare website or by calling the Medicare hotline.

Benefit period: The way that Original Medicare measures the use of hospital and skilled nursing facility (SNF) services. A benefit period begins the day a beneficiary is admitted as an inpatient in a hospital or an SNF. The benefit period ends when they haven't gotten any inpatient hospital care (or skilled care in an SNF) for sixty days in a row. If a beneficiary goes into a hospital or an SNF after one benefit period has ended, a new benefit period begins. They must pay the inpatient hospital deductible for each benefit period. There's no limit to the number of benefit periods.

- A benefit period is a set period of time during which Medicare covers certain medical services and supplies. The length of a benefit period depends on the type of service or supply being provided.

- For example, a benefit period for inpatient hospital care begins on the first day a beneficiary is formally admitted to the hospital as an inpatient and ends when they have been out of the hospital for sixty days in a row. If a beneficiary is readmitted to the hospital for a related illness within sixty days of being discharged, the new benefit period will be considered a continuation of the previous one, and they will not have to pay another inpatient deductible.

- A benefit period for SNF care begins on the first day a beneficiary receives skilled nursing care in an SNF and ends when they have not received skilled nursing care or rehabilitation services for 60 days in a row. If a beneficiary is readmitted to an SNF within thirty days of being discharged, the new benefit period will be considered a continuation of the previous one, and they will not have to pay another SNF deductible.

- It is important to note that the benefit periods described above apply only to Medicare Part A, which covers inpatient hospital and SNF care. Medicare Part B, which covers outpatient medical services and supplies, does not have benefit periods. Instead, the beneficiary is responsible for paying a copayment or coinsurance for most Part B services, and they are required to pay an annual deductible before their coverage begins.

Benefits Coordination & Recovery Center (BCRC): The company that acts on behalf of Medicare to collect and manage information on other types of insurance or coverage that a person with Medicare may have and determine whether the coverage pays before or after Medicare. This company also acts on behalf of Medicare to obtain repayment when Medicare makes a conditional payment, and the other payer is determined to be primary.

- BCRC is a division of the CMS that is responsible for coordinating the payment of benefits for Medicare beneficiaries who are also covered by other insurance plans. This may include private insurance plans, employer-sponsored plans, or state-sponsored plans such as Medicaid.

- The BCRC is responsible for ensuring that Medicare is the secondary payer for beneficiaries who have other insurance coverage, and that the other insurance plan pays its share of the beneficiary's medical bills before Medicare pays its share. The BCRC also works to recover any overpayments that may have been made by Medicare on behalf of a beneficiary.

- If a Medicare beneficiary has other insurance coverage, it is important to know that they are required to notify Medicare of their other insurance. The beneficiary can do this by completing a Medicare Secondary Payer (MSP) questionnaire and submitting it to the BCRC. This will help the BCRC determine how their benefits should be coordinated and will ensure that they receive the appropriate level of coverage.

C

Certified (Certification): See "Medicare-certified provider."

CHAMPVA: A healthcare benefit for dependents of qualifying veterans.

- CHAMPVA (Civilian Health and Medical Program of the Department of Veterans Affairs) is a healthcare program that provides coverage for certain medical services and supplies to the spouses and dependents of veterans who are permanently and totally disabled due to a service-connected disability, or who have died as a result of a service-connected disability, or who are receiving VA pension benefits.

- CHAMPVA is administered by the Department of Veterans Affairs (VA) and is a supplement to Medicare. This means that if a beneficiary is eligible for CHAMPVA and they are also enrolled in Medicare, CHAMPVA will cover certain medical expenses that are not covered by Medicare.

- CHAMPVA covers a wide range of medical services and supplies, including hospital and physician services, mental healthcare, prescription drugs, and durable medical equipment. However, it is important to note that CHAMPVA does not cover all medical expenses, and the beneficiary may be responsible for paying certain out-of-pocket costs for covered services, such as copayments, deductibles, and coinsurance.

- If a beneficiary is a spouse or dependent of a veteran who is permanently and totally disabled due to a service-connected disability, or if a beneficiary is the surviving spouse or dependent of a veteran who has died as a result of a service-connected disability, they may be eligible for CHAMPVA. To apply for CHAMPVA, the beneficiary will need to complete an application and submit it to the VA.

- If a beneficiary has any questions about CHAMPVA or their eligibility for the program, it is recommended that they contact the VA or visit the CHAMPVA website for more information.

Claim: A request for payment that a beneficiary submits to Medicare or other health insurance when they get items and services that they think are covered.

- A claim is a request for payment for medical services or supplies that a beneficiary has received. If a beneficiary is enrolled in Medicare, they or their healthcare provider may need to submit a claim to Medicare to request payment for covered services.

- There are several ways to submit a Medicare claim, depending on the type of service or supply a beneficiary has received. For example, if a beneficiary has received inpatient hospital care, their hospital will typically submit a claim to Medicare on their behalf. If a beneficiary has received outpatient medical services or supplies, their healthcare provider may submit a claim to Medicare, or they may be required to submit the claim themselves.

- It is important to note that Medicare may not cover all medical services and supplies, and a beneficiary may be responsible for paying some or all of the cost out-of-pocket. It is a good idea to discuss coverage and any potential out-of-pocket costs with a healthcare provider before receiving medical care, to ensure that a beneficiary may understand what is covered by Medicare and what they may be responsible for paying.

- If a beneficiary has any questions about submitting a Medicare claim or about their Medicare coverage, it is recommended that they contact their Medicare plan or speak with a Medicare representative.

Clinical Breast Exam: An exam by a doctor or other healthcare provider to check for breast cancer by looking for lumps or other changes. This exam isn't the same as a mammogram and is usually done in the doctor's office during a Pap test and pelvic exam.

- A clinical breast exam is a physical examination of the breasts performed by a healthcare provider. The exam is used to check for any abnormalities or changes in the breasts that may indicate the presence of breast cancer or other breast health issues.

- If an individual is enrolled in Medicare, they may be eligible to receive a clinical breast exam as part of their preventive care. Medicare covers one clinical breast exam every two years for women who are forty years of age or older and who do not have any breast symptoms or concerns.

- During a clinical breast exam, a healthcare provider will examine the breasts and surrounding areas for any lumps, swelling, or changes in the skin or nipples. The provider will also check for any discharge from the nipples and will ask about any changes or concerns the individual may have about their breasts.

- It is important to note that a clinical breast exam is not a replacement for a mammogram, which is a specialized test used to screen for breast cancer. Medicare covers mammograms for women who are forty years of age or older, and it is recommended that to discuss the appropriate frequency of mammograms with a healthcare provider.

Coinsurance: An amount a beneficiary may be required to pay as their share of the cost for services after they pay any deductibles. Coinsurance is usually a percentage (for example, 20 percent).

- Coinsurance is a type of cost-sharing that requires a beneficiary to pay a percentage of the cost of a covered medical service or supply. Coinsurance is typically a fixed percentage of the Medicare-approved amount for the service or supply and is usually required in addition to any deductibles or copayments that may be due.

- For example, if a Medicare beneficiary visits a doctor for an office visit, they may be required to pay a coinsurance of 20 percent of the Medicare-approved amount for the visit. If the Medicare-approved amount for the visit is $100, the beneficiary's coinsurance would be $20, and they would be responsible for paying that amount in addition to any applicable deductibles or copayments.

- It is important to note that Medicare coinsurance amounts can vary depending on the type of service or supply a beneficiary is receiving, as well as the specific Medicare plan they are on. Some plans may have higher or lower coinsurance amounts for certain services or may have different coinsurance amounts for inpatient and outpatient services.

Comprehensive outpatient rehabilitation facility (CORF): A facility that provides a variety of services on an outpatient basis, including physician" services, physical therapy, social or psychological services, and rehabilitation.

- A CORF is a type of medical facility that provides comprehensive outpatient rehabilitation services to individuals who have experienced a decline in physical, mental, or cognitive functioning due to illness, injury, or disability. CORFs are typically focused on providing a range of rehabilitation services, including physical therapy, occupational therapy, and speech-language therapy, to help individuals recover and improve their functional abilities.

- If a Medicare beneficiary needs rehabilitation services, they may be eligible to receive care at a CORF. Medicare covers a wide range of rehabilitation services that are provided on an outpatient basis, including those provided by a CORF.

- It is important to note that Medicare coverage for rehabilitation services may vary depending on the specific Medicare plan a beneficiary has. Some plans may have limits on the number of rehabilitation sessions that are covered or may require the beneficiary to pay a copayment or deductible for certain services. It is also important to be aware that Medicare does not cover all rehabilitation services and may not cover services that are considered experimental or investigational.

- If a beneficiary has any questions about their Medicare coverage for rehabilitation services or about CORFs, it is recommended that they contact their Medicare plan or speak with a Medicare representative. It is also a good idea to discuss their options with their healthcare provider and to consider factors such as cost, convenience, and the specific needs of their medical condition when deciding where to receive rehabilitation care.

Copayment: An amount that may be required to pay as a beneficiary's share of the cost for a medical service or supply, like a doctor's visit, hospital outpatient visit, or prescription drug. A copayment is usually a set amount, rather than a percentage. For example, a beneficiary might pay $10 or $20 for a doctor's visit or prescription drug.

- A Medicare copayment is a fixed dollar amount that a beneficiary is required to pay for a covered medical service or supply. Copayments are typically required in addition to any deductibles or coinsurance that may be due and are usually required to be paid at the time the service or supply is provided.

- For example, if a Medicare beneficiary visits a doctor for an office visit, they may be required to pay a copayment of $30 for the visit. If they visit the doctor for a different type of service, such as a laboratory test, they may be required to pay a different copayment amount.

- It is important to note that Medicare copayment amounts can vary depending on the type of service or supply a beneficiary is receiving, as well as the specific Medicare plan they have. Some plans may have higher or lower copayment amounts for certain services or may have different copayment amounts for inpatient and outpatient services.

- If a beneficiary has any questions about their Medicare copayment amounts or their Medicare coverage, it is recommended that they contact their Medicare plan or speak with a Medicare representative. It is also a good idea for a beneficiary to discuss their coverage and any potential out-of-pocket costs with their healthcare provider before receiving medical care, to ensure that they understand what is covered by Medicare and what they may be responsible for paying.

Coverage determination (Part D): The first decision made by a beneficiary's Medicare drug plan (not the pharmacy) about their drug benefits, including:

- **Whether a particular drug is covered**
- **Whether all the requirements have been met for getting a requested drug**
- **How much is required to pay for a drug**
- **Whether to make an exception to a plan rule when requested**

The drug plan must give a beneficiary a prompt decision (seventy-two hours for standard requests, twenty-four hours for expedited requests). If the beneficiary disagrees with the plan's coverage determination, the next step is an appeal.

- Coverage determination is a decision made by Medicare Part D PDP about whether a specific drug is covered under a beneficiary's plan and, if so, under what circumstances. Coverage determinations are made when the beneficiary or their healthcare provider request coverage for a prescription drug that is not included on the plan's formulary, or when the beneficiary requests an exception to a formulary rule, such as a request for a higher dosage of a covered drug.

- If a beneficiary has a Medicare Part D PDP and they have been prescribed a drug that is not covered under their plan, or if a beneficiary has been denied coverage for a drug due to a formulary rule, they have the right to request a coverage determination. To request a coverage determination, the beneficiary or their healthcare provider will need to submit a request to the plan, along with any relevant medical documentation.

- Medicare Part D plan is required to decide on the beneficiary's coverage determination request within a certain timeframe, which is specified by Medicare. If the plan denies the beneficiary's request for coverage, they have the right to appeal the decision through the Medicare Part D appeal process.

- It is important to note that coverage determinations can be complex, and it is recommended that the beneficiary seek the assistance of a healthcare professional or advocate if they are considering requesting a coverage determination or appealing a decision.

Coverage Gap: A period of time in which a beneficiary pays higher cost sharing for prescription drugs until they spend enough to qualify for catastrophic coverage. The coverage gap (also called the "donut hole") starts when the beneficiary and their plan have paid a set dollar amount for prescription drugs during that year.

- The Medicare "donut hole" is a term used to describe a coverage gap in the Medicare Part D PDP. Part D is a voluntary program that provides beneficiaries with coverage for prescription drugs. It is administered through private insurance companies and is available to Medicare beneficiaries who enroll in a Part D plan.

- Under the Part D plan, beneficiaries are responsible for paying a portion of the cost of their prescription drugs, while the plan covers the remainder. The amount that beneficiaries are required to pay is broken down into two phases, namely, the initial coverage phase and the coverage gap phase, also known as the "donut hole."

- During the initial coverage phase, beneficiaries are responsible for paying a copayment or coinsurance for their prescription drugs. Once the total cost of the drugs reaches a certain threshold, known as the "initial coverage limit," beneficiaries enter the coverage gap phase.

- In the coverage gap phase, also known as the "donut hole," beneficiaries are required to pay a higher percentage of the cost of their prescription drugs. This can be a significant financial burden for some beneficiaries, especially those who require costly medications.

- The coverage gap phase ends once the total out-of-pocket costs for the beneficiary reach a certain threshold, known as the "catastrophic coverage threshold." At this point, the beneficiary's Part

D plan begins paying for a higher percentage of the cost of their prescription drugs.

- The Medicare "donut hole" has been a controversial aspect of the Part D program since its inception. Some critics argue that it creates a financial burden for beneficiaries and may discourage them from filling their prescriptions. However, the Affordable Care Act (ACA) included several provisions to gradually close the coverage gap, and as of 2020, beneficiaries receive additional discounts on prescription drugs while in the coverage gap phase.

- Despite these efforts to reduce the financial burden of the "donut hole," it is still an important consideration for Medicare beneficiaries who are enrolled in a Part D plan. It is important for beneficiaries to understand the costs associated with their prescription drugs and to plan accordingly to avoid any unexpected expenses during the coverage gap phase.

- The MAPD "donut hole" is a term used to describe a coverage gap in the Medicare Part D PDP for beneficiaries who are enrolled in a Medicare Advantage (MA) plan. MA plans, also known as Medicare Part C, are offered by private insurance companies and provide an alternative to Original Medicare (Part A and Part B).

- Like the Part D PDP, the MAPD plan has a coverage gap, also known as the "donut hole." The coverage gap is a period during which beneficiaries are required to pay a higher percentage of the cost of their prescription drugs. This can be a significant financial burden for some beneficiaries, especially those who require costly medications.

- The MAPD coverage gap begins once the total out-of-pocket costs for the beneficiary reach a certain threshold, known as the "initial coverage limit." At this point, the beneficiary is responsible for paying a higher percentage of the cost of their prescription drugs until the total out-of-pocket costs reach a certain threshold, known as the "catastrophic coverage threshold."

- The MAPD coverage gap is similar to the Part D coverage gap, but there are some differences. For example, some MA plans may offer additional coverage, such as coverage for vision, hearing, or dental services, which are not typically covered under Original Medicare. Additionally, MA plans may have different cost-sharing requirements and may require beneficiaries to pay different copayments or coinsurance for their prescription drugs.

- It is important for beneficiaries who are enrolled in an MA plan to understand the costs associated with their prescription drugs and to plan accordingly to avoid any unexpected expenses during the MAPD coverage gap. The ACA included several provisions to gradually close the coverage gap, and beneficiaries can receive additional discounts on prescription drugs while in the coverage gap phase.

Creditable Coverage: See "creditable coverage (Medigap)" or "creditable prescription drug coverage."

- It's important to understand the concept of creditable coverage. Creditable coverage refers to health insurance that is at least as good as Original Medicare. This includes employer-sponsored insurance, individual insurance, and other types of coverage. If the beneficiary later decides to switch back to Original Medicare, they may have to pay a higher premium for Part B if they went more than sixty-three days without creditable coverage. If a beneficiary is unsure about their creditable coverage status, they can contact their insurance provider to ask whether their coverage is creditable.

- It's also a good idea to keep track of any letters received from an insurance provider about the beneficiary's creditable coverage status. These letters are called "creditable coverage disclosures," and they should be kept in a safe place in case they are needed later.

- If a beneficiary is considering switching to a Medicare Advantage plan during the Medicare Advantage Disenrollment Period (MADP), it's a good idea to speak with a Medicare advisor or an insurance provider to understand the potential consequences of losing creditable coverage. They can help make an informed decision that is right for the beneficiary.

Critical access hospital (CAH): A small facility located in a rural area more than thirty-five miles (or fifteen miles if mountainous terrain or in areas with only secondary roads) from another hospital or critical access hospital. This facility provides 24/7 emergency care, has twenty-five or fewer inpatient beds, and maintains an average length of stay of ninety-six hours or less for acute care patients.

- A CAH is a type of small, rural hospital that is designated by the CMS to provide essential healthcare services to underserved areas. CAHs are required to meet certain criteria in order to be eligible for the critical access hospital designation, including being located in a rural area, having no more than twenty-five inpatient beds, and meeting specific requirements for patient lengths of stay and services.

- If a Medicare beneficiary receives care at a critical access hospital, their Medicare coverage will generally be the same as it would be if they received care at any other hospital. This means that Medicare will cover inpatient hospital services, including room, board, and certain medical and surgical services, as well as certain outpatient services that are provided by the hospital.

- It is important to note that Medicare coverage for hospital services may vary depending on the specific Medicare plan a beneficiary has. Some plans may have limits on the number of days of hospital care that are covered or may require a copayment or deductible for certain services. It is also important to be aware that Medicare does not cover all hospital services, and the beneficiary may be responsible for paying some or all the cost out-of-pocket for certain services.

Custodial care: Nonskilled personal care, like help with activities of daily living (ADLs) like bathing, dressing, eating, getting in or out of a bed or chair, moving around, and using the bathroom. It may also include the kind of health-related care that most people do themselves, like using eye drops. In most cases, Medicare doesn't pay for custodial care.

- Custodial care refers to nonskilled, personal care services that help seniors with ADLs. Examples of custodial care include assistance with bathing, dressing, toileting, and eating.

- Custodial care is not covered by traditional Medicare (Parts A and B). This means that beneficiaries must pay out-of-pocket for these services or seek coverage through other sources, such as a long-term care insurance policy.

- However, there are some exceptions to this rule. Medicare may cover custodial care in certain situations, such as when it is provided in conjunction with skilled nursing or rehabilitation services. For example, if a beneficiary is recovering from a hip replacement surgery and needs assistance with bathing and dressing, Medicare may cover these services as part of the rehabilitation process.

- It is important for seniors to understand their coverage options for custodial care. Many seniors rely on custodial care as they age and may need to plan financially for these expenses.

- There are several ways that seniors can pay for custodial care, including:

  - Private pay: Paying for custodial care out-of-pocket.

  - Long-term care insurance: Some long-term care insurance policies cover custodial care services.

  - Medicaid: Medicaid, a joint federal and state program, may cover custodial care for low-income individuals who meet certain eligibility requirements.

- It is important for seniors to carefully consider their options and plan for potential custodial care needs as they age. Working with a certified insurance agent can help seniors understand their options and make informed decisions about their care.

D

Deductible: The amount that must be paid for healthcare or prescriptions before Original Medicare, a Medicare Advantage Plan, a Medicare drug plan, or other insurance begins to pay.

- A Medicare deductible is a set amount that a beneficiary is required to pay for covered medical services or supplies before their Medicare coverage begins to pay. Deductibles are typically required to be paid in full before the beneficiary receives any benefits and may vary depending on the type of service, or supply, they are receiving.

- For example, if a Medicare beneficiary visits a doctor for an office visit, they may be required to pay a deductible before their Medicare coverage begins to pay for the visit. If a beneficiary visits the doctor for a different type of service, such as a laboratory test, they may be required to pay a different deductible amount.

- It is important to note that Medicare deductibles can vary depending on the type of service or supply a beneficiary is receiving, as well as the specific Medicare plan they have. Some plans may have higher or lower deductibles for certain services or may have different deductibles for inpatient and outpatient services.

Demonstrations: Special projects, sometimes called "pilot programs" or "research studies," that test improvements in Medicare coverage, payment, and quality of care. They usually operate only for a limited time, for a specific group of people, and in specific areas.

- Demonstrations are pilot programs that test new approaches to providing Medicare benefits. These programs are implemented by the CMS, a federal agency within the Department of Health and Human Services (HHS).

- There are several types of demonstrations that CMS may implement, including:

  - Payment demonstrations: These test new payment models for Medicare services, such as paying for value rather than volume. The goal is to reduce costs and improve the quality of care for beneficiaries.

  - Service delivery demonstrations: These test new ways of delivering Medicare services, such as telemedicine or home-based care. The goal is to improve access to care and reduce costs.

- Quality improvement demonstrations: These test new strategies for improving the quality of care for Medicare beneficiaries, such as reducing hospital readmissions.

- CMS selects demonstrations based on their potential to improve the efficiency and effectiveness of the Medicare program. Demonstrations are typically implemented on a limited basis and may be expanded if they are successful.

- Beneficiaries may be able to participate in demonstrations if they meet certain eligibility requirements. However, participation is generally voluntary, and beneficiaries have the option to opt out if they choose.

- Overall, demonstrations play an important role in shaping the future of the Medicare program. They allow CMS to test new approaches and gather data on their effectiveness, which can inform policy decisions and help improve the quality of care for beneficiaries.

Diethylstilbestrol: A drug given to pregnant women from the early 1940s until 1971 to help with common problems during pregnancy. The drug has been linked to cancer of the cervix or vagina in women whose mother took the drug while pregnant.

Donut Hole: See "Coverage Gap"

Durable Medical Equipment (DME): Certain medical equipment, like a walker, wheelchair, or hospital bed, that's ordered by a doctor for use in the home.

- DME is a category of medical equipment that is used to provide medical or therapeutic benefits to a patient and that can withstand repeated use. Examples of DME include wheelchairs, hospital beds, oxygen tanks, and blood sugar monitors.

- If a Medicare beneficiary has a need for DME, their Medicare coverage will generally depend on the specific type of DME they are using and the medical condition it is being used to treat. Medicare generally covers DME that is medically necessary and meets certain criteria, such as being used in the treatment of a Medicare-covered condition and being prescribed by a Medicare-approved healthcare provider.

- It is important to note that Medicare coverage for DME may vary depending on the specific Medicare plan a beneficiary has. Some plans may have limits on the number of covered DME items or may require the beneficiary to pay a copayment or deductible for certain items. It is also important to be aware that Medicare does not cover all types of DME, and the beneficiary may be responsible for paying some or all the cost out-of-pocket for certain items.

- If a beneficiary has any questions about their Medicare coverage for DME or about the types of DME that are covered by Medicare, it is recommended that they contact their Medicare plan or speak with a Medicare representative. The beneficiary may also want to discuss their DME needs and coverage with their healthcare provider to ensure that they understand what is covered and what they may be responsible for paying.

Durable power of attorney (DPOA): A legal document that names someone else to make healthcare decisions for an individual. This is helpful if a person becomes unable to make their own decisions.

- A durable power of attorney (DPOA) is a legal document that allows an individual to appoint someone else, known as an "agent," to make decisions on the behalf of the individual in the event that they are unable to make decisions for themself. A DPOA can be used to make financial, legal, and healthcare decisions, and can take effect immediately or at a specific time in the future, such as when the individual becomes incapacitated or unable to make decisions due to illness or injury.

- If an individual is enrolled in Medicare and has a DPOA, it is important to be aware that their agent may be able to make decisions on their behalf regarding their Medicare coverage and healthcare. This may include deciding which Medicare plan to enroll in, selecting a primary care provider, or making decisions about medical treatment.

- It is important to note that a DPOA is a legal document that must be signed and witnessed according to the individual's state's laws. It is a good idea to discuss a DPOA with a healthcare professional or an attorney to ensure that it meets the state's requirements and that it accurately reflects wishes of the individual.

- If an individual has any questions about durable powers of attorney or about their Medicare coverage, it is recommended that they speak with a healthcare professional or an attorney. They may also want to contact their Medicare plan or speak with a Medicare representative for more information.

E

End-Stage Renal Disease (ESRD): Permanent kidney failure that requires a regular course of dialysis or a kidney transplant.

- ESRD is a medical condition in which the kidneys are no longer able to function effectively, resulting in the build-up of waste products in the body. ESRD typically requires dialysis or a kidney transplant to sustain life.

- If a Medicare beneficiary has ESRD, Medicare has a special program, known as the ESRD Program, that provides coverage for dialysis and kidney transplant services for individuals with ESRD.

- Under the ESRD Program, Medicare covers a variety of services related to ESRD, including inpatient and outpatient dialysis, kidney transplants, and certain medical supplies and equipment. The specific services that are covered and the costs that are associated with these services can vary depending on the type of service a beneficiary is receiving, and the specific Medicare plan they have.

- It is important to note that Medicare coverage for ESRD services is generally limited to those that are medically necessary and that are provided by Medicare-approved providers. It is a good idea to review Medicare coverage and discuss treatment options with a healthcare provider to ensure that a beneficiary understands what is covered and what they may be responsible for paying.

Exception: A type of Medicare prescription drug coverage determination. A formulary exception is a drug plan's decision to cover a drug that's not on its drug list or to waive a coverage rule. A tiering exception is a drug plan's decision to charge a lower amount for a drug that's on its nonpreferred drug tier. The beneficiary or their prescriber must request an exception, and their doctor or other prescriber must provide a supporting statement explaining the medical reason for the exception.

- Medicare drug exceptions are typically made in situations where an individual has a medical need for a prescription drug that is not covered by the individual's PDP, but where the drug is deemed medically necessary by the individual's healthcare provider.

- To request a Medicare drug exception, a beneficiary will need to submit a written request to their PDP explaining their medical need for the drug and providing supporting documentation from their healthcare provider. The beneficiary's PDP will review their request and decide about whether to grant the exception. If the request is granted, the beneficiary's PDP may provide coverage for the drug either through a coverage determination or through a formulary exception.

- It is important to note that Medicare drug exceptions are not guaranteed, and a request may be denied if it is not deemed medically necessary or if it does not meet other Medicare coverage criteria. If a request for a Medicare drug exception is denied, the beneficiary may have the option to appeal the decision.

Excess charge: If an individual has Original Medicare, and the amount a doctor or other healthcare provider is legally permitted to charge is higher than the Medicare-approved amount, the difference is called the excess charge.

- An excess charge is a charge for a Medicare-covered service or item that is above the amount that is approved by Medicare. Medicare excess charges are generally not allowed under the Medicare program, with a few exceptions.

- If a Medicare beneficiary receives a service or item that is covered by the program, they are generally required to pay the Medicare-approved amount for the service or item. This is known as the "Medicare-approved amount" or the "Medicare rate." If a beneficiary receives a service or item that is covered by Medicare and they are charged more than the Medicare-approved amount, they may be responsible for paying the excess charge out-of-pocket.

- There are a few exceptions to the rule against Medicare excess charges. For example, if a beneficiary sees a healthcare provider who does not accept assignment (meaning that the provider does not agree to accept the Medicare-approved amount as payment in full), the provider may charge up to 15 percent more than the Medicare-approved amount for a service. In this case, the beneficiary may be responsible for paying the excess charge out-of-pocket.

- It is important to note that Medicare excess charges can vary depending on the type of service or item a beneficiary is receiving, and the specific Medicare plan they have. If a beneficiary has any questions about their Medicare coverage or about excess charges, it is recommended that they contact their Medicare plan or speak with a Medicare representative. The beneficiary may also want to discuss their coverage with their healthcare provider to ensure that they understand what is covered and what they may be responsible for paying.

Extra Help: A Medicare program to help people with limited income and resources pay Medicare prescription drug program costs, like premiums, deductibles, and coinsurance.

- Extra Help is a program that provides financial assistance to Medicare beneficiaries who have limited income and resources and who are enrolled in a Medicare PDP. The Medicare Extra Help program is also known as the Low-Income Subsidy (LIS) program.

- If a Medicare beneficiary is eligible for the Medicare Extra Help program, they may be able to receive help paying for prescription drug premiums, deductibles, and copayments. The specific amount of assistance the beneficiary receives will depend on their income and resources, as well as the specific Medicare PDP they are enrolled in.

- To be eligible for the Medicare Extra Help program, a beneficiary must meet certain income and resource limits.

- If a beneficiary believes that they may be eligible for the Medicare Extra Help program, it is recommended that they contact the

Social Security Administration (SSA) to apply for the program. The beneficiary can apply for the Medicare Extra Help program online at the SSA website, by calling the SSA at 1-800-772-1213, or by visiting a local SSA office.

- If a beneficiary has any questions about the Medicare Extra Help program or about their eligibility for the program, it is recommended that they contact the SSA or speak with a Medicare representative. The beneficiary may also want to discuss their coverage with their healthcare provider to ensure that they understand what is covered and what they may be responsible for paying.

F

Formulary: A list of prescription drugs covered by a prescription drug plan or another insurance plan offering prescription drug benefits. Also called a drug list.

- A Medicare formulary is a list of prescription drugs that are covered under a Medicare PDP. Medicare formularies vary depending on the specific PDP a beneficiary is enrolled in and may include drugs that are covered by the plan, as well as any restrictions or limitations on coverage.

- If a beneficiary is enrolled in a Medicare PDP, it is important to be aware of the formulary for their plan. The formulary can help a beneficiary understand what prescription drugs are covered by their plan and what costs they may be responsible for paying for these drugs. For example, a formulary may include information about whether the beneficiary is required to pay a copayment or deductible for a prescription drug, or whether there are any limits on the number of prescriptions that can be filled for a particular drug.

- It is important to note that Medicare formularies can change from year to year, and a PDP may add or remove drugs from the formulary or change the cost-sharing requirements for certain drugs. If a beneficiary is taking a prescription drug that is covered by their PDP, it is a good idea to review the formulary each year to ensure that the drug is still covered and to understand any changes to the cost-sharing requirements.

- If a beneficiary has any questions about their Medicare formulary or about their prescription drug coverage, it is recommended that they contact their PDP or speak with a Medicare representative. The beneficiary may also want to discuss their coverage with their healthcare provider to ensure that they understand the treatment options and any potential out-of-pocket costs.

G

Grievance: A complaint about the way a beneficiary's Medicare health plan or Medicare drug plan is giving care. For example, a beneficiary may file a grievance if they have a problem calling the plan or if they are unhappy with the way a staff person at the plan has behaved toward them. However, if a beneficiary has a complaint about a plan's refusal to cover a service, supply, or prescription, they need to file an appeal.

- A grievance is a complaint or concern that a beneficiary has about the quality of care or services that was received through their Medicare plan. Medicare grievances can be about a wide range of issues, including concerns about the treatment a beneficiary received, problems with their healthcare provider or facility, or issues with their Medicare coverage or benefits.

- If a Medicare beneficiary has a grievance about the care or services received, they have the right to file a grievance with their Medicare plan. To file a grievance, a beneficiary will need to contact their Medicare plan and explain the issue they are concerned about. The beneficiary's Medicare plan is required to investigate the grievance and provide a written response.

- It is important to note that Medicare grievances are different from Medicare appeals, which are requests for Medicare to review a decision that has been made about a beneficiary's coverage or payment for a service or item. If the beneficiary is dissatisfied with a decision that has been made by their Medicare plan and they believe that the decision is incorrect, an appeal may be filed instead of a grievance.

- If a beneficiary has any questions about filing a Medicare grievance or about their Medicare coverage or benefits, it is recommended that to contact the Medicare plan or speak with a Medicare representative. The beneficiary may also want to discuss their concerns with their healthcare provider to ensure that they understand their treatment options and any potential out-of-pocket costs.

Group Health Plan: In general, a health plan offered by an employer or employee organization that provides health coverage to employees and their families.

- A group health plan is a type of health insurance plan that is offered by an employer or other group, such as a union or professional organization, to its employees or members. Group health plans typically provide coverage for a wide range of healthcare services, including doctor's visits, hospital stays, and prescription drugs.

- If a Medicare beneficiary has coverage through a group health plan, their Medicare coverage may be different from the coverage that is available to other beneficiaries. This is because Medicare works with certain types of group health plans to coordinate benefits and help ensure that beneficiaries receive the most appropriate care at the lowest cost to them.

- The way in which a beneficiary's Medicare coverage works with their group health plan will depend on the specific type of group health plan they have. For example, if a beneficiary has an "employer-sponsored" group health plan, that plan is required to pay for certain services before Medicare does. In this case, Medicare may pay for certain services that are not covered by the group health plan, or it may pay for services that are covered by the plan but that have a cost-sharing requirement, such as a copayment or deductible.

- If a beneficiary has any questions about how their group health plan works with their Medicare coverage, it is recommended that they contact their group health plan or speak with a Medicare representative. The beneficiary may also want to discuss the coverage with their healthcare provider to ensure that they understand the treatment options and any potential out-of-pocket costs.

Guaranteed Issue Rights (also called "Medigap Protections"): Rights a beneficiary has in certain situations when insurance companies are required by law to sell or offer a Medigap policy. In these situations, an insurance company can't deny the beneficiary a Medigap policy, or place conditions on a Medigap policy, like exclusions for pre-existing conditions, and can't charge more for a Medigap policy because of a past or present health problem.

- Guaranteed issue rights, also known as "Medigap protections," refer to the rights that Medicare beneficiaries have to purchase a Medicare Supplement Insurance (Medigap) policy without being denied coverage or charged more due to a pre-existing medical condition.

- If a Medicare beneficiary is interested in purchasing a Medigap policy, in certain situations, they have guaranteed issue rights that allow the purchase of a policy without being denied coverage or charged more due to medical history. These rights apply to certain situations, such as when a beneficiary first becomes eligible for Medicare, when coverage is lost through an employer or group health plan, or when a beneficiary moves out of the service area of their current Medigap policy.

- It is important to note that guaranteed issue rights do not apply in all situations, and a beneficiary may not be eligible for these rights if they have had a Medigap policy in the past and let it expire or if they are eligible for a Medicare Advantage plan. In these cases, the beneficiary may be required to undergo medical underwriting, which means that the Medigap insurer can consider their medical history when deciding whether to offer coverage and at what price.

- If a beneficiary has any questions about their guaranteed issue rights or about purchasing a Medigap policy, it is recommended that they contact a Medigap insurer or speak with a Medicare representative. The beneficiary may also want to discuss their coverage options with their healthcare provider to ensure that they understand the treatment options and any potential out-of-pocket costs.

Guaranteed Renewable Policy: An insurance policy that can't be terminated by the insurance company unless a beneficiary makes untrue statements to the insurance company, commits fraud, or doesn't pay the premiums. All Medigap policies issued since 1992 are guaranteed renewable.

- A guaranteed renewable policy is a type of insurance policy that is guaranteed to be renewed by the insurer, as long as the policyholder continues to pay the required premiums.

- Medicare Supplement Insurance (Medigap) policies are an example of guaranteed renewable policies. If a Medicare beneficiary has a Medigap policy, the policy is guaranteed to be renewed by the insurer as long as premium payments are made on time. This means that the insurer cannot cancel the policy due to any changes to the beneficiary's health.

- It is important to note that guaranteed renewable policies may still be subject to certain limitations or exclusions. For example, a Medigap policy may not cover certain medical services or may have exclusions for pre-existing conditions. It is a good idea for a beneficiary to review the policy carefully to understand what is and is not covered, and to discuss coverage with their healthcare provider to ensure that they understand the treatment options and any potential out-of-pocket costs.

- If a beneficiary has any questions about their Medigap policy or about their Medicare coverage, it is recommended that they contact the Medigap insurer or speak with a Medicare representative. The beneficiary may also want to discuss their coverage with their healthcare provider to ensure that they understand the treatment options and any potential out-of-pocket costs.

H

Healthcare Provider: A person or organization that's licensed to give healthcare. Doctors, nurses, and hospitals are examples of healthcare providers.

- A healthcare provider is a healthcare professional or facility that is approved to provide services to Medicare beneficiaries. Medicare healthcare providers may include doctors, hospitals, nursing homes, home health agencies, and other types of providers that are enrolled in the Medicare program.

- If a Medicare beneficiary is seeking healthcare services, it is important to make sure that the provider they are seeing is a Medicare healthcare provider. This is because Medicare will only cover services that are provided by Medicare-approved providers. If a beneficiary receives services from a provider who is not approved by Medicare, they may be responsible for paying for those services out-of-pocket.

- To find a Medicare healthcare provider, a beneficiary can use the Medicare website or call the Medicare hotline at 1-800-MEDICARE (1-800-633-4227). A beneficiary can also ask their healthcare provider for recommendations or consult with a healthcare professional, such as a doctor or nurse, to find providers who are approved by Medicare.

- If a beneficiary has any questions about finding a Medicare healthcare provider or about their Medicare coverage, it is recommended that they contact Medicare or speak with a Medicare representative. The beneficiary may also want to discuss their coverage with their healthcare provider to ensure that they understand the treatment options and any potential out-of-pocket costs.

Health Insurance Marketplace: A service that helps people shop for and enroll in affordable health insurance. The federal government operates the Marketplace, available at HealthCare.gov, for most states. Some states run their own Marketplaces. The Health Insurance Marketplace (also known as the "Marketplace" or "exchange") provides health plan shopping and enrollment services through websites, call centers, and in-person help.

- The Health Insurance Marketplace, also known as the Medicare Exchange, is a website that allows Medicare beneficiaries to compare and enroll in Medicare Advantage plans and Medicare Part D PDPs. The Medicare Health Insurance Marketplace is operated by the CMS and is available to all Medicare beneficiaries who are eligible to enroll in a Medicare Advantage plan or a PDP.

- If a Medicare beneficiary is interested in exploring coverage options, they can use the Medicare Health Insurance Marketplace to compare different plans and enroll in a plan that best meets their needs. When using the Marketplace, a beneficiary will be able to compare plans based on factors such as premiums, deductibles, copayments, and covered benefits. They will also be able to see whether a plan has any restrictions or limitations on coverage.

- To use the Medicare Health Insurance Marketplace, a beneficiary will need to create an account and provide some basic information, such as their Medicare number and their zip code. After an account has been created, the beneficiary will be able to browse available plans and enroll in a plan online.

- If a beneficiary has any questions about the Medicare Health Insurance Marketplace or about Medicare coverage options, it is recommended that they visit the Marketplace website or speak with a Medicare representative. The beneficiary may also want to discuss their coverage with their healthcare provider to ensure that they understand the treatment options and any potential out-of-pocket costs.

Home Health Agency: An organization that provides home healthcare.

- A home health agency is an organization that provides in-home healthcare services to Medicare beneficiaries. Home health agencies are typically licensed and certified by Medicare to provide a range of services, including nursing care, physical therapy, occupational therapy, and home health aide services.

- If a Medicare beneficiary needs in-home healthcare services, they may be eligible to receive services from a Medicare home health agency. To be eligible for home health services through Medicare, a beneficiary must be homebound (meaning they are unable to leave their home without significant difficulty), and they must be under the care of a doctor. The beneficiary must also be receiving services from a home health agency that is approved by Medicare.

- To receive services from a Medicare home health agency, a beneficiary will need to have a face-to-face visit with a healthcare professional (such as a doctor or nurse practitioner) who will determine eligibility for home health services. If the beneficiary is eligible, the healthcare professional will create a plan of care that outlines the services that they will receive and the frequency of those services.

- If a beneficiary has any questions about receiving services from a Medicare home health agency or about their Medicare coverage, it is recommended that they contact a home health agency or speak with a Medicare representative. The beneficiary may also want to discuss their coverage with their healthcare provider to ensure that they understand the treatment options and any potential out-of-pocket costs.

Home Healthcare: A broad range of healthcare services that can be given in your home for an injury or illness.

- Home healthcare is a type of medical care that is provided to individuals in their own homes. It is typically used for people who are unable to leave their homes due to a medical condition or disability, and who need ongoing medical treatment or rehabilitation.

- One of the main benefits of Medicare home healthcare is that it allows individuals to receive high-quality medical care while still maintaining their independence and the comfort of their own home. This can be especially important for older adults or those with chronic conditions who may not have the mobility or energy to travel to a medical facility for treatment.

- Medicare home healthcare services are typically provided by a team of healthcare professionals, including doctors, nurses, therapists, and other specialists. The specific types of services provided will depend on the individual's needs and may include things like wound care, medication management, physical therapy, occupational therapy, and more.

- To be eligible for Medicare home healthcare, individuals must meet certain criteria. For example, they must be under the care of a doctor and have a medical condition that requires ongoing treatment or rehabilitation. In addition, they must be home-bound, which means that it is medically necessary for them to be at home, and it would be difficult for them to leave their home due to their medical condition.

- Medicare covers a wide range of home healthcare services, including medical and rehabilitation services, as well as medical equipment and supplies. However, it is important to note that there may be some limitations on coverage, and some services may not be covered at all. It is always a good idea to check with Medicare or a healthcare provider to find out what is covered and what is not.

- Medicare home healthcare is a valuable resource for individuals who need ongoing medical treatment or rehabilitation, but who are unable to leave their homes due to a medical condition or disability. With the help of a team of healthcare professionals, individuals can receive the care they need to maintain their health and independence, all from the comfort of their own home.

Hospice: A special way of caring for people who are terminally ill. Hospice care involves a team-oriented approach that addresses the medical, physical, social, emotional, and spiritual needs of the patient. Hospice also provides support to the patient's family or caregiver.

- Hospice is a type of medical care that is provided to individuals who are facing a terminal illness and who have a life expectancy of six months or less. The goal of hospice care is to help individuals live as comfortably as possible during their final months and to provide support and resources to their families and caregivers.

- One of the main benefits of Medicare hospice is that it focuses on providing comfort and symptom management, rather than attempting to cure the terminal illness. This can allow individuals to spend their remaining time in a peaceful and comfortable environment, surrounded by loved ones.

- Medicare hospice care is typically provided by a team of healthcare professionals, including doctors, nurses, therapists, and other specialists. The specific types of services provided will depend on the individual's needs and may include things like pain management, symptom control, spiritual support, and more.

- To be eligible for Medicare hospice, individuals must meet certain criteria. For example, they must be under the care of a doctor and have a terminal illness with a life expectancy of six months or less. In addition, they must choose to forgo curative treatment for their terminal illness and instead opt for hospice care.

- Medicare covers a wide range of hospice services, including medical and support services, as well as medical equipment and supplies. However, it is important to note that there may be some limitations on coverage, and some services may not be covered at all. It is always a good idea to check with Medicare or a healthcare provider to find out what is covered and what is not.

- Medicare hospice is a valuable resource for individuals who are facing a terminal illness and who want to focus on comfort and symptom management during their final months. With the help of a team of healthcare professionals, individuals can receive the support and resources they need to live as comfortably as possible, surrounded by loved ones.

I

Income Related Monthly Adjustment Amount (IRMAA): IRMAA is an additional amount that is added to the beneficiaries Part B and Part D monthly premiums for individuals who had a modified adjusted gross income that exceeded a certain amount. The IRMAA is based on a beneficiary's income as reported on their tax return from two years.

Independent reviewer: An organization (sometimes called an Independent Review Entity or IRE) that has no connection to a Medicare health plan or Medicare Prescription Drug Plan. Medicare contracts with the IRE to review a case if a beneficiary appeals their plan's payment or coverage decision or if the plan doesn't make a timely appeals decision.

- Independent reviewers are healthcare professionals who are responsible for reviewing medical claims and making decisions about whether or not they should be covered by Medicare. They play a crucial role in the Medicare system, as they help to ensure that the medical treatment and services provided to beneficiaries are necessary, appropriate, and cost-effective.

- One of the main benefits of Medicare independent reviewers is that they are not affiliated with any particular healthcare provider or medical facility. This means that they are able to make unbiased decisions about what should and should not be covered by Medicare.

- There are several types of Medicare independent reviewers, including medical review nurses, medical review physicians, and an administrative law judge. The specific role of an independent reviewer will depend on the type of medical claim being reviewed and the individual's area of expertise.

- Medicare independent reviewers may be called upon to review a wide range of medical claims, including claims for hospital stays, outpatient procedures, DME, and more. They will consider factors such as the individual's medical history, the proposed treatment or service, and the potential benefits and risks of the treatment or service.

- To be eligible for review by a Medicare independent reviewer, an individual's medical claim must meet certain criteria. For example, the claim must have been denied by Medicare, or the individual must have requested an appeal of the decision. In addition, the individual must have exhausted all other available avenues of appeal before turning to an independent reviewer.

- Medicare independent reviewers are healthcare professionals who play a crucial role in the Medicare system by reviewing medical claims and making decisions about what should and should not be covered. They are able to provide unbiased decisions, ensuring that the medical treatment and services provided to beneficiaries are necessary, appropriate, and cost-effective.

Initial Coverage Election Period (ICEP): The ICEP is a one-time event that occurs three months before the beneficiary becomes eligible for both Part A and Part B. During this period, the beneficiary also becomes eligible for a Medicare Advantage Plan (Part C).

Initial Enrollment Period (IEP): This is a seven-month period when beneficiaries first enroll in Medicare. The IEP includes your sixty-fifth birthday month, the three months before and the three months after.

Inpatient Rehabilitation Facility: A hospital, or part of a hospital, that provides an intensive rehabilitation program to inpatients.

- Inpatient rehabilitation facilities (IRFs) are medical facilities that provide intensive, multidisciplinary rehabilitation services to individuals who have had a serious illness or injury. The goal of IRF care is to help individuals regain their strength, mobility, and independence, so that they can return to their homes and communities as quickly and safely as possible.

- One of the main benefits of Medicare IRF care is that it is provided by a team of healthcare professionals, including doctors, nurses, therapists, and other specialists. This allows individuals to receive the comprehensive care and support they need to make a full recovery.

- Medicare IRFs provide a wide range of rehabilitation services, including physical therapy, occupational therapy, speech-language therapy, and more. The specific types of services provided will depend on the individual's needs and may include things like muscle re-education, functional training, and pain management.

- To be eligible for Medicare IRF care, individuals must meet certain criteria. For example, they must be under the care of a doctor and have a medical condition that requires intensive rehabilitation. In addition, they must be expected to make significant progress toward their goals within a reasonable amount of time, and they must require the intensive rehabilitation services that are only available in an IRF.

- Medicare covers a wide range of IRF services, including medical and rehabilitation services, as well as medical equipment and supplies. However, it is important to note that there may be some limitations on coverage, and some services may not be covered at all. It is always a good idea to check with Medicare or a healthcare provider to find out what is covered and what is not.

- Medicare inpatient rehabilitation facilities are medical facilities that provide intensive, multidisciplinary rehabilitation services to individuals who have had a serious illness or injury. With the help of a team of healthcare professionals, individuals can receive the comprehensive care and support they need to make a full recovery and return to their homes and communities.

J

No Content

K

No Content

L

Large Group Health Plan: In general, a group health plan that covers employees of either an employer or employee organization that has at least 100 employees.

- A large group health plan is a type of health insurance that is provided to employees of large companies or organizations. It is typically offered as part of an employee benefit package and can cover a wide range of medical expenses, including hospital stays, outpatient procedures, and prescription medications.

- One of the main benefits of a large group health plan is that it can provide employees with access to high-quality medical care at an affordable price. Large group plans are often able to negotiate lower rates with healthcare providers, which can result in lower out-of-pocket costs for employees.

- For individuals who are enrolled in Medicare, a large group health plan can work in conjunction with their Medicare coverage to provide additional benefits and protections. For example, a large group health plan may cover services that are not covered by Medicare, or it may provide additional financial assistance for deductibles and copays.

- It is important to note that large group health plans are subject to different rules and regulations than individual or small group health plans. For example, they are not required to follow the same enrollment periods as individual plans and may have different rules for pre-existing conditions.

- A large group health plan is a type of health insurance that is provided to employees of large companies or organizations. It can work in conjunction with Medicare to provide additional benefits and protections and can help individuals access high-quality medical care at an affordable price. However, it is important to understand the specific rules and regulations that apply to large group health plans.

Lifetime Reserve Days: In Original Medicare, these are additional days that Medicare will pay for when a beneficiary is in a hospital for more than ninety days. A beneficiary has a total of sixty reserve days that can be used during their lifetime. For each lifetime reserve day, Medicare pays all covered costs except for daily coinsurance.

- Lifetime reserve days are a type of coverage that is available to individuals who are enrolled in Medicare Part A (hospital insurance). These days are intended to provide additional protection in the event of a prolonged hospital stay or other medical emergency and can be used when an individual has exhausted their standard Medicare coverage.

- One of the main benefits of Medicare lifetime reserve days is that they can provide individuals with the financial protection they need to cover the costs of a prolonged hospital stay or other medical emergency. This can be especially important for individuals who have a high risk of developing a serious illness or injury, or who have a preexisting medical condition.

- Medicare lifetime reserve days can be used in addition to an individual's standard Medicare Part A coverage. Each individual has a total of sixty lifetime reserve days that they can use throughout their lifetime. These days can be used in blocks of up to sixty days at a time and can be used at any point during the individual's Medicare coverage.

- It is important to note that Medicare lifetime reserve days are not free, and individuals will be responsible for paying a daily coinsurance amount for each day that they use their reserve days. The specific coinsurance amount will depend on the individual's Medicare Part A deductible and other factors.

- Medicare lifetime reserve days are a type of coverage that is available to individuals who are enrolled in Medicare Part A. These days can provide additional protection in the event of a prolonged hospital stay or other medical emergency and can be used when an individual has exhausted their standard Medicare coverage. However, it is important to understand that there is a cost associated with using these days.

Limiting Charge : In Original Medicare, the highest amount of money a beneficiary can be charged for a covered service by doctors and other healthcare suppliers who don't accept assignment. The limiting charge is 15 percent over Medicare's approved amount. The limiting charge only applies to certain services and doesn't apply to supplies or equipment.

- Limiting charges are a type of financial protection that is available to individuals who are enrolled in Medicare Part B (medical insurance). These charges are intended to limit the amount of money that an individual has to pay out-of-pocket for certain medical services and supplies and are designed to protect individuals from being charged excessive fees by healthcare providers.

- One of the main benefits of Medicare limiting charges is that they can help individuals to manage their healthcare costs and avoid unexpected financial surprises. This can be especially important for individuals who have a high risk of developing a serious illness or injury, or who have a preexisting medical condition.

- Medicare limiting charges apply to certain medical services and supplies that are provided by Medicare-participating providers. These providers are required to accept the Medicare limiting charge as payment in full for these services and supplies, and they are not allowed to charge the individual any additional fees.

- It is important to note that Medicare limiting charges do not apply to all medical services and supplies, and there may be situations in which an individual is responsible for paying a larger out-of-pocket cost. For example, limiting charges may not apply to services that are provided by nonparticipating providers, or to services that are not medically necessary.

Living Will: A written legal document, also called a "medical directive" or "advance directive." It shows what type of treatments an individual wants or doesn't want in case they can't speak for themself, like whether the individual wants life support. Usually, this document only comes into effect if an individual is unconscious.

- A living will is a legal document that allows individuals to express their wishes for end-of-life medical care in the event that they are unable to make decisions for themselves. It is an important tool for ensuring that an individual's wishes are respected and followed, even if they are unable to communicate them.

- One of the main benefits of a living will is that it can provide individuals with peace of mind, knowing that their wishes for end-of-life medical care will be followed. This can be especially important for individuals who are enrolled in Medicare, as it can help to ensure that their Medicare coverage is used in a way that is consistent with their wishes.

- A living will is typically created with the help of a lawyer or other legal professional, and it should be signed and witnessed by two individuals who are not related to the individual creating the will. The living will should include specific instructions about the individual's wishes for end-of-life medical care, such as whether they want to be kept on life support, receive pain medication, or undergo certain medical procedures.

- It is important to note that a living will is not the same as a DPOA for healthcare, which is a legal document that allows an individual to appoint someone else to make medical decisions on their behalf. A living will only goes into effect if the individual is unable to make their own decisions, whereas a DPOA for healthcare can be used at any time.

Long-Term Care: Services that include medical and nonmedical care provided to people who are unable to perform basic activities of daily living (ADL), like dressing or bathing. Long-term support and services can be provided at home, in the community, in assisted living, or in nursing homes. Individuals may need long-term support and services at any age. Medicare and most health insurance plans don't pay for long-term care.

- Long-term care is a type of medical care that is provided to individuals who are unable to perform everyday tasks due to a chronic illness or disability. It is typically used for people who need ongoing assistance with these activities and can include things like nursing home care, assisted living, and in-home care.

- One of the main benefits of long-term care is that it can help individuals to maintain their independence and quality of life, even if they are unable to perform everyday tasks on their own. This can be especially important for older adults or those with chronic conditions who may need ongoing support and assistance.

- For individuals who are enrolled in Medicare, long-term care can be a complex and confusing topic. Medicare does not generally cover long-term care services, with a few exceptions. For example, Medicare may cover a limited amount of SNF care or home healthcare for certain individuals who meet certain criteria.

- It is important to note that there are other options available for paying for long-term care, such as private insurance, Medicaid, or out-of-pocket payments. These options can vary significantly in terms of coverage, eligibility requirements, and cost, and it is important to carefully consider all of the available options before making a decision.

- ADLs are basic self-care tasks that individuals need to complete on a daily basis in order to maintain their independence and quality of life. ADLs include activities such as:

  - Eating/Feeding (the ability of a person to feed oneself)
  - Bathing
  - Dressing (the ability to select appropriate clothes and to put the clothes on)
  - Personal hygiene (the ability to bathe and groom oneself and maintain dental hygiene, nail, and hair care)
  - Continence (the ability to control bladder and bowel function)
  - Toileting (the ability to get to and from the toilet, using it appropriately, and cleaning oneself)
  - Transferring/Ambulating (the extent of an individual's ability to move from one position to another and walk independently)

- The ability to complete ADLs is an important factor in determining an individual's need for long-term care. As people age or experience a decline in their health, they may need assistance with ADLs in order to continue living safely and independently.

- There are several types of long-term care services that can help individuals with ADLs, including:

- Home care: Home care services provide assistance with ADLs in the individual's home. This can include help with bathing, dressing, and other self-care tasks, as well as light housekeeping and meal preparation.

- Assisted living: Assisted living facilities provide housing and support services for seniors who need assistance with ADLs. These facilities may offer a range of services, including help with bathing, dressing, and other self-care tasks, as well as meals, transportation, and social activities.

- Skilled nursing facilities: Skilled nursing facilities, also known as nursing homes, provide twenty-four-hour medical supervision and assistance with ADLs for individuals who are unable to live independently. These facilities may offer rehabilitation services and specialized care for individuals with chronic medical conditions.

- Long-term care insurance is one option for paying for long-term care services, including those that help with ADLs. Medicare and Medicaid may also cover some long-term care services, but coverage is limited to skilled care and eligibility requirements vary.

- It is important for individuals to plan for their long-term care needs as they age, as the cost of these services can be significant. Working with a certified insurance agent can help individuals understand their options and make informed decisions about their care.

Long-Term Care Hospital: Acute care hospitals that provide treatment for patients who stay, on average, more than twenty-five days. Most patients are transferred from an intensive or critical care unit. Services provided include comprehensive rehabilitation, respiratory therapy, head trauma treatment, and pain management.

- A long-term care hospital (LTCH) is a type of medical facility that provides specialized care to individuals who are critically ill and require a longer hospital stay than what is typically provided in a traditional hospital. LTCHs are designed to provide intensive, specialized care to patients who have complex medical needs, and who are expected to make significant progress toward their goals within a reasonable amount of time.

- One of the main benefits of a long-term care hospital is that it can provide individuals with the specialized care and support they need to make a full recovery. This can be especially important for individuals who have a serious illness or injury and who require a longer hospital stay than what is typically provided in a traditional hospital.

- For individuals who are enrolled in Medicare, long-term care hospitals are an important resource for obtaining the specialized care and support they need to make a full recovery. Medicare covers a wide range of services provided by long-term care hospitals, including medical and rehabilitation services, as well as medical equipment and supplies.

- It is important to note that there may be some limitations on Medicare coverage for long-term care hospitals, and some services may not be covered at all. It is always a good idea to check with Medicare or a healthcare provider to find out what is covered and what is not.

Long-Term Care Ombudsman: An independent advocate (supporter) for nursing home and assisted living facility residents who works to solve problems of residents of nursing homes, assisted living facilities, or similar facilities. They may be able to provide information about home health agencies in their area.

- A long-term care ombudsman is a trained and certified individual who advocates for the rights and well-being of individuals who are receiving long-term care. Ombudsmen are trained to help individuals understand their rights and options and to assist them in resolving any issues or concerns they may have about their care.

- One of the main benefits of a long-term care ombudsman is that they can provide individuals with the support and resources they need to navigate the long-term care system and advocate for themselves. This can be especially important for individuals who are enrolled in Medicare, as they may have questions or concerns about their coverage and care.

- Long-term care ombudsmen are available to assist individuals in a variety of settings, including nursing homes, assisted living facilities, and in-home care. They can provide assistance with a wide range of issues, such as complaints about the quality of care, questions about coverage and billing, and more.

- It is important to note that long-term care ombudsmen are independent advocates and are not affiliated with any particular long-term care provider or government agency. They are able to provide unbiased assistance and support to individuals and can help ensure that their rights and well-being are protected.

M

Medicaid: A joint federal and state program that helps with medical costs for some people with limited income and resources. Medicaid programs vary from state to state, but most healthcare costs are covered if an individual qualifies for both Medicare and Medicaid.

- Medicaid is a government-funded healthcare program that provides medical coverage to low-income individuals and families.

It is administered by the states and is designed to help those who are unable to afford private health insurance or who do not have access to employer-sponsored coverage.

- One of the main benefits of Medicaid is that it can provide individuals with access to high-quality medical care at an affordable price. Medicaid covers a wide range of medical services, including hospital stays, outpatient procedures, and prescription medications, and can help individuals to manage their healthcare costs and stay healthy.

- For individuals who are enrolled in Medicare, Medicaid can work in conjunction with their Medicare coverage to provide additional benefits and protections. For example, Medicaid may cover services that are not covered by Medicare, or it may provide additional financial assistance for deductibles and copays.

- It is important to note that Medicaid eligibility and coverage can vary significantly from state to state, and individuals may need to meet certain income and asset requirements to be eligible for coverage. In addition, Medicaid may not cover all medical services and supplies, and there may be limitations on coverage.

Medical Underwriting: The process that an insurance company uses to decide, based on an individual's medical history, whether to take an application for insurance, whether to add a waiting period for pre-existing conditions (if a state law allows it), and how much to charge for that insurance.

- Medical underwriting is the process by which insurers assess an individual's health status and risk for developing certain medical conditions in order to determine their eligibility for coverage and the premiums they will be charged. Medical underwriting is typically used by private health insurers and is not typically used by Medicare.

- One of the main benefits of medical underwriting is that it can help insurers to accurately assess an individual's risk for developing certain medical conditions, which can help ensure that they are able to provide coverage at an affordable price. However, medical underwriting can also have some drawbacks, as it can result in individuals being denied coverage or charged higher premiums based on their health status.

- For individuals who are enrolled in Medicare, medical underwriting is generally not a concern, as Medicare does not use medical underwriting to determine eligibility or premiums. Instead, Medicare uses a system of standardized premiums and deductibles that are based on factors such as age, income, and geographic location.

- It is important to note that while Medicare does not use medical underwriting, there are certain situations in which an individual may be required to undergo medical underwriting in order to obtain coverage. For example, an individual who is applying for a Medigap plan may be required to undergo medical underwriting in order to determine their eligibility and premiums.

Medically Necessary: Healthcare services or supplies needed to diagnose or treat an illness, injury, condition, disease, or its symptoms and that meet accepted standards of medicine.

- Medically necessary services are healthcare services or supplies that are deemed necessary by a healthcare provider to diagnose, treat, or prevent an illness or injury. These services are considered essential for maintaining an individual's health and well-being and are generally covered by Medicare.

- One of the main benefits of medically necessary services is that they can help individuals to access the care and treatment they need to manage their health and maintain their quality of life. This can be especially important for individuals who are enrolled in Medicare, as Medicare covers a wide range of medically necessary services and supplies.

- Medicare covers a wide range of medically necessary services, including hospital stays, outpatient procedures, and prescription medications. In order for a service to be considered medically necessary and covered by Medicare, it must be ordered by a healthcare provider, be reasonable and necessary for the diagnosis or treatment of an illness or injury and meet certain other criteria.

- It is important to note that there may be some limitations on Medicare coverage for medically necessary services, and some services may not be covered at all. It is always a good idea to check with Medicare or a healthcare provider to find out what is covered and what is not.

Medicare: Medicare is the federal health insurance program for:

- **People who are sixty-five or older**
- **Certain younger people with disabilities**
- **People with End-Stage Renal Disease (permanent kidney failure requiring dialysis or a transplant, sometimes called ESRD)**

- Medicare is a government-funded healthcare program that provides medical coverage to individuals who are sixty-five years of age or older, or to those who are under sixty-five and have certain disabilities or conditions such as ESRD or Lou Gehrig's disease. Medicare is administered by the CMS and is designed to help individuals access the medical care they need to maintain their health and well-being.

- There are several different parts to Medicare, including:

  - Part A: Hospital insurance that covers inpatient hospital stays, nursing facility care, hospice care, and some home healthcare services.

  - Part B: Medical insurance that covers certain outpatient medical services, such as doctor visits, preventive care, and medical equipment.

  - Part C: Medicare Advantage plans that are offered by private insurance companies and provide coverage for the services covered under Part A and Part B, as well as additional benefits.

  - Part D: Prescription drug coverage that helps individuals to pay for the cost of prescription medications.

- One of the main benefits of Medicare is that it can help individuals to access the medical care they need to maintain their health and well-being. It covers a wide range of medical services and supplies and can help individuals to manage their healthcare costs and stay healthy.

- It is important to note that Medicare does not cover all medical services and supplies, and there may be limitations on coverage. In addition, individuals may be responsible for paying premiums, deductibles, and copays for certain services.

Medicare Advantage Plan (Part C): A type of Medicare health plan offered by a private company that contracts with Medicare. Medicare Advantage Plans provide all of Part A and Part B benefits, with a few exclusions, for example, certain aspects of clinical trials which are covered by Original Medicare even though a beneficiary is still in the plan. Medicare Advantage Plans include:

- Health Maintenance Organizations
- Preferred Provider Organizations
- Private Fee-for-Service Plans
- Special Needs Plans
- Medicare Medical Savings Account Plans

If a beneficiary is enrolled in a Medicare Advantage Plan:

- Most Medicare services are covered through the plan
- Most Medicare services aren't paid for by Original Medicare
- Most Medicare Advantage Plans offer prescription drug coverage
- Medicare Advantage Plans, also known as Part C, are a type of Medicare plan that is offered by private insurance companies. These plans are designed to provide coverage for the services covered under Original Medicare (Parts A and B), as well as additional benefits such as vision, dental, and hearing coverage.
- One of the main benefits of Medicare Advantage Plans is that they can provide individuals with access to a wide range of medical services and benefits all in one place. These plans often have lower out-of-pocket costs than Original Medicare and may also include additional benefits such as routine vision, dental, and hearing coverage.

- There are several different types of Medicare Advantage Plans, including Health Maintenance Organizations (HMOs), Preferred Provider Organizations (PPOs), Private Fee-for-Service (PFFS) plans, and Special Needs Plans (SNPs). Each type of plan has its own unique features and benefits, and it is important to carefully consider all of the available options before enrolling.

- It is important to note that Medicare Advantage Plans are required to provide at least the same level of coverage as Original Medicare, but they may have different rules and restrictions on coverage. In addition, individuals who enroll in a Medicare Advantage Plan may be required to use certain healthcare providers or facilities in order to receive coverage.

Medicare Cost Plan: A type of Medicare health plan available in some areas. In a Medicare Cost Plan, if a beneficiary receives services outside of the plan's network without a referral, the Medicare-covered services will be paid for under Original Medicare (the Cost Plan pays for emergency services or urgently needed services).

- A Medicare Cost Plan is a type of Medicare plan that is offered by private insurance companies. These plans are designed to provide coverage for the services covered under Original Medicare (Parts A and B), as well as additional benefits such as vision, dental, and hearing coverage.

- One of the main benefits of a Medicare Cost Plan is that it can provide individuals with access to a wide range of medical services and benefits all in one place. These plans often have lower out-of-pocket costs than Original Medicare and may also include additional benefits such as routine vision, dental, and hearing coverage.

- Medicare Cost Plans are available in certain areas of the country and may be a good option for individuals who live in areas where other Medicare plan options are not available. It is important to note that Medicare Cost Plans are required to provide at least the same level of coverage as Original Medicare, but they may have different rules and restrictions on coverage.

- In addition, Medicare Cost Plans may not be available in all areas, and individuals who enroll in a Medicare Cost Plan may be required to use certain healthcare providers or facilities in order to receive coverage. It is always a good idea to carefully consider all of the available Medicare plan options before enrolling.

Medicare Drug Coverage (Part D): Optional benefits for prescription drugs available to all people with Medicare for an additional charge. This coverage is offered by insurance companies and other private companies approved by Medicare.

- Medicare drug coverage, also known as Part D, is a Medicare benefit that helps individuals to pay for the cost of prescription medications. It is administered by private insurance companies that have been approved by Medicare and is designed to help individuals access the medications they need to maintain their health and well-being.

- One of the main benefits of Medicare drug coverage is that it can help individuals to manage the cost of their prescription medications. It covers a wide range of medications, including both generic and brand-name drugs, and can help individuals to save money on their medications.

- There are several different types of Medicare drug plans available, including stand-alone PDPs and Medicare Advantage plans with prescription drug coverage (MA-PDs). Each type of plan has its own unique features and benefits, and it is important to carefully consider all of the available options before enrolling.

- It is important to note that Medicare drug coverage has certain rules and restrictions on coverage, and not all medications are covered. In addition, individuals may be responsible for paying premiums, deductibles, and copays for their drug coverage.

Medicare Drug Plan (Part D): Part D adds prescription drug coverage to:

- **Original Medicare**
- **Some Medicare Cost Plans**
- **Some Medicare Private-Fee-for-Service Plans**
- **Medicare Medical Savings Account Plans**

These plans are offered by insurance companies and other private companies approved by Medicare. Medicare Advantage Plans may also offer prescription drug coverage that follows the same rules as Medicare drug plans.

- A Medicare drug plan (Part D) is a Medicare benefit that helps individuals to pay for the cost of prescription medications. It is administered by private insurance companies that have been approved by Medicare and is designed to help individuals access the medications they need to maintain their health and well-being.

- One of the main benefits of a Medicare drug plan is that it can help individuals to manage the cost of their prescription medications. It covers a wide range of medications, including both generic and brand-name drugs, and can help individuals to save money on their medications.

- There are several different types of Medicare drug plans available, including stand-alone PDPs and MA-PDs. Each type of plan has its own unique features and benefits, and it is important to carefully consider all of the available options before enrolling.

- It is important to note that Medicare drug plans have certain rules and restrictions on coverage, and not all medications are covered. In addition, individuals may be responsible for paying premiums, deductibles, and copays for their drug coverage.

Medicare Health Maintenance Organization (HMO) Plan: A type of Medicare Advantage Plan (Part C) available in some areas of the country. In most HMOs, beneficiaries can only go to doctors, specialists, or hospitals on the plan's list except in an emergency. Most HMOs also require a beneficiary to get a referral from their primary care physician.

- A Medicare Health Maintenance Organization (HMO) Plan is a type of Medicare Advantage Plan that is offered by private insurance companies. These plans are designed to provide coverage for the services covered under Original Medicare (Parts A and B), as well as additional benefits such as vision, dental, and hearing coverage.

- One of the main benefits of a Medicare HMO Plan is that it can provide beneficiaries with access to a wide range of medical services and benefits all in one place. These plans often have lower out-of-pocket costs than Original Medicare and may also include additional benefits such as routine vision, dental, and hearing coverage.

- Medicare HMO Plans typically require beneficiaries to choose a primary care physician and to get a referral from that physician in order to see a specialist. These plans may also have a limited network of healthcare providers and facilities that beneficiaries can use in order to receive coverage.

- It is important to note that Medicare HMO Plans are required to provide at least the same level of coverage as Original Medicare, but they may have different rules and restrictions on coverage. In addition, individuals who enroll in a Medicare HMO Plan may be required to use certain healthcare providers or facilities in order to receive coverage.

Medicare Health Plan: Generally, a plan offered by a private company that contracts with Medicare to provide Part A and Part B benefits to people with Medicare who enroll in the plan. Medicare health plans include all Medicare Advantage Plans, Medicare Cost Plans, and Demonstration/Pilot Programs. Program of All-inclusive Care for the Elderly (PACE) organizations are special types of Medicare health plans. PACE plans can be offered by public or private companies and provide Part D and other benefits in addition to Part A and Part B benefits.

- A Medicare health plan is a type of insurance plan that is designed to provide coverage for the medical services and benefits covered under Medicare. There are several different types of Medicare health plans available, including Original Medicare (Parts A and B), Medicare Advantage Plans (Part C), and Medicare Cost Plans.

- One of the main benefits of a Medicare health plan is that it can help individuals to access the medical care and benefits they need to maintain their health and well-being. These plans can provide coverage for a wide range of medical services and supplies, including hospital stays, outpatient procedures, and prescription medications.

- It is important to note that each type of Medicare health plan has its own unique features and benefits, and it is important to carefully consider all of the available options before enrolling. In addition, Medicare health plans may have certain rules and restrictions on coverage, and individuals may be responsible for paying premiums, deductibles, and copays for certain services.

Medicare Medical Savings Account (MSA) Plan: MSA Plans combine a high deductible Medicare Advantage Plan and a bank account. The plan deposits money from Medicare into the account. A beneficiary can use the money in this account to pay for their healthcare costs, but only Medicare-covered expenses count toward their deductible. The amount deposited is usually less than the deductible amount so a beneficiary generally will have to pay out-of-pocket before their coverage begins.

- A Medicare MSA Plan is a type of Medicare Advantage Plan that combines a high deductible health plan with a personal savings account. These plans are designed to provide coverage for the services covered under Original Medicare (Parts A and B), as well as additional benefits such as vision, dental, and hearing coverage.

- One of the main benefits of a Medicare MSA Plan is that it can provide individuals with access to a wide range of medical services and benefits all in one place. These plans often have lower premiums than other Medicare Advantage Plans, and the money in the personal savings account can be used to pay for covered medical expenses.

- It is important to note that Medicare MSA Plans have certain rules and restrictions on coverage, and individuals may be responsible for paying higher deductibles and copays for certain services. In addition, the money in the personal savings account must be used within a certain timeframe, and any money that is not used may be forfeited.

Medicare Part A (Hospital Insurance): Part A covers inpatient hospital stays, care in a skilled nursing facility, hospice care, and some home healthcare.

- Medicare Part A (Hospital Insurance) is a Medicare benefit that helps individuals to pay for the cost of inpatient hospital stays, nursing facility care, hospice care, and some home healthcare services. It is designed to help individuals access the medical care they need to maintain their health and well-being.

- One of the main benefits of Medicare Part A is that it can help individuals to manage the cost of hospital stays and other inpatient medical services. It covers a wide range of services, including inpatient hospital stays, nursing facility care, hospice care, and some home healthcare services.

- It is important to note that Medicare Part A has certain rules and restrictions on coverage, and individuals may be responsible for paying premiums, deductibles, and copays for certain services. In addition, Medicare Part A only covers certain types of inpatient medical services, and it does not cover outpatient services or prescription medications.

Medicare Part B (Medical Insurance): Part B covers certain doctors' services, outpatient care, medical supplies, and preventive services.

- Medicare Part B (Medical Insurance) is a Medicare benefit that helps beneficiaries to pay for certain outpatient medical services, such as doctor visits, preventive care, and medical equipment. It is designed to help beneficiaries access the medical care they need to maintain their health and well-being.

- One of the main benefits of Medicare Part B is that it can help beneficiaries to manage the cost of outpatient medical services. It covers a wide range of services, including doctor visits, preventive care, and medical equipment.

- It is important to note that Medicare Part B has certain rules and restrictions on coverage, and beneficiaries may be responsible for paying premiums, deductibles, and copays for certain services. In addition, Medicare Part B only covers certain types of outpatient medical services, and it does not cover inpatient hospital stays or prescription medications.

Medicare Plan: Any way other than Original Medicare that a beneficiary can get their Medicare health or drug coverage. This term includes all Medicare health plans and Medicare drug plans.

- A Medicare plan is a type of insurance plan that is designed to provide coverage for the medical services and benefits covered under Medicare. There are several different types of Medicare plans available, including Original Medicare (Parts A and B), Medicare Advantage Plans (Part C), and Medicare Cost Plans.

- One of the main benefits of a Medicare plan is that it can help individuals to access the medical care and benefits they need to maintain their health and well-being. These plans can provide coverage for a wide range of medical services and supplies, including hospital stays, outpatient procedures, and prescription medications.

- It is important to note that each type of Medicare plan has its own unique features and benefits, and it is important to carefully consider all of the available options before enrolling. In addition, Medicare plans may have certain rules and restrictions on coverage, and individuals may be responsible for paying premiums, deductibles, and copays for certain services.

Medicare Preferred Provider Organization (PPO) Plan: A type of Medicare Advantage Plan (Part C) available in some areas of the country in which a beneficiary pays less if they use doctors, hospitals, and other healthcare providers that belong to the plan's network. Beneficiaries can use doctors, hospitals, and providers outside of the network for an additional cost.

- A Medicare Preferred Provider Organization (PPO) Plan is a type of Medicare Advantage Plan that is offered by private insurance companies. These plans are designed to provide coverage for the services covered under Original Medicare (Parts A and B), as well as additional benefits such as vision, dental, and hearing coverage.

- One of the main benefits of a Medicare PPO Plan is that it can provide beneficiaries with access to a wide range of medical services and benefits all in one place. These plans often have lower out-of-pocket costs than Original Medicare and may also include additional benefits such as routine vision, dental, and hearing coverage.

- Medicare PPO Plans typically allow beneficiaries to see any healthcare provider that accepts Medicare, although they may have lower out-of-pocket costs if they use providers within the plan's network. These plans may also have deductibles, copays, and coinsurance for certain services.

- It is important to note that Medicare PPO Plans are required to provide at least the same level of coverage as Original Medicare, but they may have different rules and restrictions on coverage. In addition, individuals who enroll in a Medicare PPO Plan may be responsible for paying premiums in addition to their Part B premium.

Medicare Private Fee-For-Service (PFFS) Plan: A type of Medicare Advantage Plan (Part C) in which a beneficiary can generally go to any doctor or hospital an individual could go to if they had Original Medicare, if the doctor or hospital agrees to treat them. The plan determines how much it will pay doctors and hospitals, and how much the beneficiary must pay when they get care. A Private Fee-For-Service Plan is very different than Original Medicare, and a beneficiary must follow the plan rules carefully when they go for healthcare services. When a beneficiary is in a Private Fee-For-Service Plan, they may pay more or less for Medicare-covered benefits than in Original Medicare.

- A Medicare Private Fee-For-Service (PFFS) Plan is a type of Medicare Advantage Plan that is offered by private insurance companies. These plans are designed to provide coverage for the services covered under Original Medicare (Parts A and B), as well as additional benefits such as vision, dental, and hearing coverage.

- One of the main benefits of a Medicare PFFS Plan is that it can provide individuals with access to a wide range of medical services and benefits all in one place. These plans often have lower out-of-pocket costs than Original Medicare and may also include additional benefits such as routine vision, dental, and hearing coverage.

- Medicare PFFS Plans typically allow individuals to see any healthcare provider that accepts the terms and conditions of the plan, although they may have lower out-of-pocket costs if they use providers within the plan's network. These plans may also have deductibles, copays, and coinsurance for certain services.

- It is important to note that Medicare PFFS Plans are required to provide at least the same level of coverage as Original Medicare, but they may have different rules and restrictions on coverage.

In addition, individuals who enroll in a Medicare PFFS Plan may be responsible for paying premiums in addition to their Part B premium.

Medicare Savings Program: A Medicaid program that helps people with limited income and resources pay some or all of their Medicare premiums, deductibles, and coinsurance.

- Medicare Savings Programs are state assistance programs that help individuals with low income and limited assets to pay for their Medicare premiums, deductibles, and copays. There are several different types of Medicare Savings Programs available, including the Qualified Medicare Beneficiary (QMB) Program, the Specified Low-Income Medicare Beneficiary (SLMB) Program, and the Qualifying Individual (QI) Program.

- One of the main benefits of a Medicare Savings Program is that it can help individuals with low income and limited assets to afford their Medicare coverage. These programs are designed to provide financial assistance to individuals who may otherwise be unable to afford their Medicare premiums, deductibles, and copays.

- To be eligible for a Medicare Savings Program, individuals must be enrolled in Medicare and have a low income and limited assets. Each state has its own eligibility requirements for these programs, and individuals may be required to provide documentation of their income and assets in order to qualify.

- It is important to note that Medicare Savings Programs are administered by the states, and the specific benefits and eligibility requirements may vary from state to state. In addition, these programs are subject to change, and individuals should regularly review their eligibility and benefit levels to ensure that they are still receiving the appropriate level of assistance.

Medicare SELECT: A type of Medigap policy that may require a beneficiary to use hospitals and, in some cases, doctors within its network to be eligible for full benefits.

- Medicare SELECT is a type of Medicare Supplement Insurance (Medigap) policy that is offered by private insurance companies. These policies are designed to provide coverage for the out-of-pocket costs that are not covered by Original Medicare (Parts A and B), such as deductibles, copays, and coinsurance.

- One of the main benefits of Medicare SELECT is that it can provide individuals with additional coverage for their medical expenses. These policies are designed to help individuals to manage the out-of-pocket costs associated with their Medicare coverage and can provide coverage for a wide range of medical services and supplies.

- It is important to note that Medicare SELECT policies have certain rules and restrictions on coverage, and individuals may be required to use specific providers in order to receive benefits. In addition, these policies may have deductibles, copays, and coinsurance for certain services.

Medicare Special Needs Plan (SNP): A special type of Medicare Advantage Plan (Part C) that provides more focused and specialized healthcare for specific groups of people, like those who have both Medicare and Medicaid, who live in a nursing home, or have certain chronic medical conditions.

- A Medicare Special Needs Plan (SNP) is a type of Medicare Advantage Plan that is designed to provide targeted care for specific populations of Medicare beneficiaries. These plans are available to individuals who meet certain eligibility criteria, such as those who have certain chronic conditions, live in a nursing home, or are dually eligible for Medicare and Medicaid.

- One of the main benefits of a Medicare SNP is that it can provide individuals with access to a wide range of medical services and benefits that are tailored to their specific needs. These plans often have lower out-of-pocket costs than Original Medicare and may also include additional benefits such as routine vision, dental, and hearing coverage.

- Medicare SNPs typically allow individuals to see any healthcare provider that accepts Medicare, although they may have lower out-of-pocket costs if they use providers within the plan's network. These plans may also have deductibles, copays, and coinsurance for certain services.

- It is important to note that Medicare SNPs are required to provide at least the same level of coverage as Original Medicare, but they may have different rules and restrictions on coverage. In addition, individuals who enroll in a Medicare SNP may be responsible for paying premiums in addition to their Part B premium.

Medicare Summary Notice (MSN): A notice a beneficiary receives after the doctor, other healthcare provider, or supplier files a claim for Part A or Part B services in Original Medicare. It explains what the doctor, other healthcare provider, or supplier billed for, the Medicare-approved amount, how much Medicare paid, and what the beneficiary must pay.

- An MSN is a document that is mailed to Medicare beneficiaries to provide information about their Medicare claims and benefits. It is designed to help individuals understand their Medicare coverage and out-of-pocket costs and to identify any potential errors or discrepancies in their claims.

- One of the main benefits of an MSN is that it can help individuals to stay informed about their Medicare coverage and out-of-pocket costs. It provides a summary of the medical services and supplies that were billed to Medicare, as well as any deductibles, copays, and coinsurance that were applied. It also includes information about the remaining benefits available under the individual's Medicare coverage.

- It is important to note that individuals should review their MSN carefully, and to report any errors or discrepancies to their Medicare provider. If an individual disagrees with a claim decision, they have the right to appeal the decision through the Medicare appeals process.

Medicare-Approved Amount: In Original Medicare, this is the amount a doctor or supplier that accepts assignment can be paid. It may be less than the actual amount a doctor or supplier charges. Medicare pays part of this amount, and the beneficiary is responsible for the difference.

- The Medicare-approved amount is the amount that Medicare will pay for a covered medical service or item. This amount is determined by Medicare and is based on a variety of factors, such as the type of service or item, the location where it is provided, and any applicable Medicare policies or guidelines.

- One of the main benefits of the Medicare-approved amount is that it helps ensure that individuals receive high-quality medical care at a reasonable cost. By setting a standard amount for covered services and items, Medicare can help control healthcare costs and ensure that individuals are not charged excessively for their care.

- It is important to note that the Medicare-approved amount is not necessarily the same as the amount that an individual will be required to pay for a covered service or item. In many cases, individuals may be responsible for paying deductibles, copays, and coinsurance in addition to the Medicare-approved amount.

Medicare-Certified Provider: A healthcare provider (like a home health agency, hospital, nursing home, or dialysis facility) that's been approved by Medicare. Providers are approved or "certified" by Medicare if they've passed an inspection conducted by a state government agency. Medicare only covers care given by providers who are certified.

- A Medicare-certified provider is a healthcare provider or facility that has met the requirements for participating in the Medicare program. These providers have agreed to follow the terms and conditions of the Medicare program, including the Medicare benefit policies and payment rules.

- One of the main benefits of using a Medicare-certified provider is that individuals can be assured that they are receiving high-quality medical care that meets the standards set by Medicare. These providers are required to meet certain qualifications and standards in order to participate in the Medicare program, which helps ensure that they are capable of providing high-quality care to their patients.

- It is important to note that Medicare-certified providers are not the same as Medicare providers. Medicare providers are healthcare providers or facilities that have enrolled in the Medicare program but have not necessarily been certified by Medicare.

Medigap: Medicare Supplement Insurance sold by private insurance companies to fill "gaps" in Original Medicare coverage.

- Medigap, also known as Medicare Supplement Insurance, is a type of private insurance that is designed to supplement Original Medicare (Parts A and B). These policies are offered by private insurance companies and are designed to cover the out-of-pocket costs that are not covered by Original Medicare, such as deductibles, copays, and coinsurance.

- One of the main benefits of Medigap is that it can help individuals to manage the out-of-pocket costs associated with their Medicare coverage. These policies are designed to provide additional coverage for medical expenses and can help individuals to afford the cost of their care.

- It is important to note that Medigap policies have certain rules and restrictions on coverage, and individuals may be required to use specific providers in order to receive benefits. In addition, these policies may have deductibles, copays, and coinsurance for certain services.

Medigap Open Enrollment Period: A one-time only, six-month period when federal law allows beneficiaries to buy any Medigap policy they want that's sold in their state. It starts in the first month covered under Part B and the beneficiary is age sixty-five years or older. During this period, a beneficiary can't be denied a Medigap policy or charged more due to past or present health problems. Some states may have additional open enrollment rights under state law.

- The Medigap Open Enrollment Period is a six-month period during which individuals who are enrolled in Original Medicare (Parts A and B) are allowed to purchase a Medigap policy without having to undergo medical underwriting. This period begins the month that an individual is sixty-five years old and enrolled in Medicare Part B.

- One of the main benefits of the Medigap Open Enrollment Period is that it allows individuals to purchase a Medigap policy without having to worry about being denied coverage due to pre-existing conditions. During this period, insurance companies are required to sell a Medigap policy to any individual who is eligible, regardless of their health status.

- It is important to note that the Medigap Open Enrollment Period is a limited-time opportunity, and individuals who miss this window may have to undergo medical underwriting in order to purchase a Medigap policy. In addition, Medigap policies may not be available to individuals who are under the age of sixty-five or who are not enrolled in Medicare Part B.

Medigap policy: Medicare Supplement Insurance sold by private insurance companies to fill "gaps" in Original Medicare coverage.

- Medigap, also known as Medicare Supplement Insurance, is a type of private insurance that is designed to supplement Original Medicare (Parts A and B). These policies are offered by private insurance companies and are designed to cover the out-of-pocket costs that are not covered by Original Medicare, such as deductibles, copays, and coinsurance.

- One of the main benefits of Medigap is that it can help individuals to manage the out-of-pocket costs associated with their Medicare coverage. These policies are designed to provide additional coverage for medical expenses and can help individuals to afford the cost of their care.

- It is important to note that Medigap policies have certain rules and restrictions on coverage, and individuals may be required to use specific providers in order to receive benefits. In addition, these policies may have deductibles, copays, and coinsurance for certain services.

Multi-employer plan: In general, a group health plan that's sponsored jointly by two or more employers.

- A multi-employer health plan is a type of group health insurance plan that is jointly sponsored by multiple employers and a labor union. These types of plans are commonly found in industries with a high number of unionized workers, such as construction and manufacturing.

- One of the main benefits of a multi-employer health plan is that it allows participating employees to move between employers within the same industry and still maintain their health insurance coverage. This can be particularly beneficial for workers who may not have a long tenure with a single employer.

- In a multi-employer health plan, the participating employers and the labor union work together to negotiate the terms of the plan with insurance carriers. This can often result in more favorable rates for plan participants compared to what they might be able to secure on their own as an individual.

- It's important to note that not all multi-employer health plans are the same, and it's important for participants to carefully review the terms of their plan to understand what is covered and any potential limitations.

- Overall, multi-employer health plans can be a valuable source of healthcare coverage for unionized workers and can provide a level of stability and security for workers who may move between employers within the same industry.

N

No Content

O

Open Enrollment Period (OEP): The OEP period begins January 1st and ends on March 31st. During the OEP, an existing Medicare Advantage policyholder can switch their Medicare advantage plan and/or cancel their enrollment in their Medicare Advantage plan to return to Original Medicare and enroll in a Medicare Part D plan.

Original Medicare: Original Medicare is a fee-for-service health plan that has two parts: Part A (Hospital Insurance) and Part B (Medical Insurance). After a deductible is paid, Medicare pays its share of the Medicare-approved amount, and the beneficiary pays their share (coinsurance and deductibles).

- Original Medicare is the federally funded healthcare program that provides coverage for millions of seniors and disabled individuals in the United States. It is administered by the CMS and consists of two main parts: Part A (hospital insurance) and Part B (medical insurance).

- Part A of Original Medicare covers inpatient hospital care, SNF care, hospice care, and some home healthcare services. Part B covers outpatient medical services, such as doctor's visits, preventive care, and some home healthcare services.

- One of the key features of Original Medicare is that it is a fee-for-service program, which means that beneficiaries pay a deductible and copayment for each service received. There are also limits on how much Medicare will pay for certain services, and beneficiaries may be responsible for paying any remaining costs out of pocket.

- While Original Medicare provides a wide range of coverage, it does not cover everything. For example, it does not cover most prescription drugs, dental care, or long-term care. Beneficiaries can choose to purchase a separate Medicare Part D plan to cover prescription drugs, and they may also consider purchasing a Medicare supplement (Medigap) policy to help cover some of the out-of-pocket costs associated with Original Medicare.

- Overall, Original Medicare is an important source of healthcare coverage for seniors and disabled individuals, but it is important for beneficiaries to understand its limitations and consider whether additional coverage may be necessary to meet their healthcare needs.

Out-Of-Pocket Costs: Health or prescription drug costs that a beneficiary must pay because they aren't covered by Medicare or other insurance.

- Out-of-pocket costs are expenses that are not covered by an insurance plan and are the responsibility of the individual to pay. In the context of Medicare, out-of-pocket costs can include deductibles, copayments, and coinsurance for covered services.

- Under Original Medicare (consisting of Part A and Part B), beneficiaries are responsible for paying a deductible for each benefit period. A benefit period begins when a beneficiary is admitted to the hospital and ends when they have not received inpatient care for sixty consecutive days.

- After the deductible has been met, Medicare Part A covers most inpatient hospital care. Medicare Part B has a yearly deductible, after which it covers most covered services at 80 percent, with beneficiaries responsible for paying the remaining 20 percent coinsurance.

- Overall, it's important for Medicare beneficiaries to understand their out-of-pocket costs and consider whether a MAPD plan, Medigap policy or a Medicare Part D plan may be necessary to help cover these expenses and provide additional financial protection.

P

Pap Test: A test to check for cancer of the cervix, the opening to a woman's uterus. It's done by removing cells from the cervix. The cells are then prepared so they can be seen under a microscope.

- A Pap test, also known as a Pap smear, is a screening test that is used to detect abnormal cells in the cervix, which is the lower part of the uterus that opens into the vagina. Pap tests are an important tool in the early detection and prevention of cervical cancer.

- Under Original Medicare, Pap tests are typically covered as a preventive service when received at regular intervals as recommended by a healthcare provider. This means that Medicare will cover the cost of the Pap test without requiring the beneficiary to pay a deductible or copayment.

- It's important to note that the specific recommendations for Pap test intervals may vary based on factors such as a beneficiary's age, medical history, and previous test results. It's important for beneficiaries to follow the recommendations of their healthcare provider in order to ensure timely screening and early detection of any potential issues.

- In addition to Pap tests, Original Medicare also covers other preventive services, such as flu shots and mammograms, at no cost to the beneficiary. It's important for beneficiaries to take advantage of these preventive services in order to maintain good health and catch any potential issues early on.

- Overall, Pap tests are an important tool in the early detection and prevention of cervical cancer, and Original Medicare covers these tests as a preventive service at no cost to the beneficiary. It's important for beneficiaries to follow the recommendations of their healthcare provider and take advantage of these preventive services.

Pelvic Exam: An exam to check if internal female organs are normal by feeling their shape and size.

- A pelvic exam is a physical examination of the female reproductive system, including the cervix, uterus, fallopian tubes, and ovaries. Pelvic exams are commonly performed by healthcare providers as part of a routine gynecological examination or as part of a diagnostic evaluation for a specific medical concern.

- Under Original Medicare, pelvic exams are generally covered as medically necessary services when ordered by a healt-care provider. This means that Medicare will cover the cost of the exam, subject to any applicable deductibles and copayments.

- It's important to note that the specific recommendations for pelvic exams may vary based on factors such as a beneficiary's age, medical history, and symptoms. It's important for beneficiaries to follow the recommendations of their healthcare provider in order to ensure timely evaluation and treatment of any potential issues.

- In addition to pelvic exams, Original Medicare also covers a wide range of other diagnostic and treatment services, including laboratory tests, X-rays, and surgeries. It's important for beneficiaries to understand the terms of their coverage and any potential out-of-pocket costs that may be involved.

- Overall, pelvic exams are an important tool in the evaluation and treatment of a range of medical concerns, and Original Medicare covers these exams as medically necessary services when ordered by a healthcare provider. It's important for beneficiaries to follow the recommendations of their healthcare provider and understand their coverage.

Penalty: An amount added to the monthly premium for Part B or a Medicare drug plan (Part D) if a beneficiary didn't join when they were first eligible. The beneficiary pays this higher amount as long as they have Medicare. There are some exceptions.

- Penalties in the context of Medicare refer to additional costs that may be incurred by beneficiaries who do not take certain actions or meet certain requirements. There are several types of penalties that may be applicable to Medicare beneficiaries, including the following:

- Late enrollment penalty: If a beneficiary does not enroll in Medicare Part B (medical insurance) during their initial enrollment period and decides to enroll at a later date, they may be subject to a late enrollment penalty. This penalty is a permanent increase in the Part B premium and is based on the number of months that the beneficiary was eligible for Part B but did not enroll.

- Part D late enrollment penalty: Similar to the Part B late enrollment penalty, beneficiaries who do not enroll in a Medicare Part D (prescription drug) plan during their initial enrollment period and decide to enroll at a later date may be subject to a late enrollment penalty. This penalty is also a permanent increase in the Part D premium and is based on the number of months that the beneficiary was without creditable prescription drug coverage.

- It's important for Medicare beneficiaries to understand the potential penalties that may apply to them and to take steps to avoid incurring them. This may include enrolling in Medicare during the initial enrollment period, maintaining creditable prescription drug coverage, and understanding the terms of their Medicare coverage.

Pilot Programs: See "Demonstrations."

Point-Of-Service Option: In a Health Maintenance Organization (HMO), this option allows beneficiaries use doctors and hospitals outside the plan for an additional cost.

- A point-of-service (POS) option is a type of Medicare Advantage plan that allows beneficiaries to receive healthcare services from a provider outside of the plan's network, although they may be subject to higher out-of-pocket costs for doing so.

- Medicare Advantage plans are private health insurance plans that are approved by Medicare and are an alternative to Original Medicare (consisting of Part A and Part B). These plans must cover everything that Original Medicare covers, but they may offer additional benefits and have different out-of-pocket costs.

- POS plans typically have a network of providers that beneficiaries can choose from, and they may offer lower out-of-pocket costs when services are received from in-network providers. However, beneficiaries also have the option of receiving care from out-of-network providers, although they may be subject to higher out-of-pocket costs for doing so.

- It's important for beneficiaries to carefully review the terms of their POS plan and understand the potential out-of-pocket costs for using out-of-network providers. In some cases, it may be more cost-effective for a beneficiary to receive care from an in-network provider, even if it means traveling a greater distance.

- Overall, POS plans can offer beneficiaries flexibility in their choice of healthcare providers, but it's important for beneficiaries to understand the potential costs associated with using out-of-network providers.

Power of attorney: A medical power of attorney is a document that lets an individual appoint someone they trust to make decisions about their medical care. This type of advance directive also may be called a healthcare proxy, appointment of healthcare agent, or a durable power of attorney for healthcare.

- A power of attorney (POA) is a legal document that allows an individual to appoint someone else, known as an "agent," to act on their behalf in financial or medical matters. A power of attorney can be useful in a variety of situations, including if an individual becomes incapacitated or otherwise unable to manage their own affairs.

- In the context of Medicare, a power of attorney can be particularly useful for beneficiaries who may not have someone else, such as a spouse or family member, who can act on their behalf. A POA allows the beneficiary to appoint an agent to make decisions about their Medicare coverage and healthcare treatment, if necessary.

- It's important for beneficiaries to carefully consider their choice of agent and to clearly communicate their wishes and preferences with regards to their Medicare coverage and healthcare treatment. The POA should be properly executed and properly witnessed, and a copy should be given to the agent and kept in a safe place.

- It's also important for beneficiaries to understand that a power of attorney is not the same as a healthcare power of attorney or living will, which are separate legal documents that allow individuals to specify their healthcare treatment preferences in the event that they are unable to make decisions for themselves.

- Overall, a power of attorney can be a useful tool for Medicare beneficiaries to ensure that their affairs are properly managed in the event that they are unable to do so themselves. It's important for beneficiaries to carefully consider their choice of agent and to clearly communicate their wishes and preferences.

Pre-Existing Condition: A health problem an individual had before the date that new health coverage starts.

- A pre-existing condition is a medical condition that an individual had before enrolling in a health insurance plan. Under certain circumstances, insurance plans may exclude coverage for treatment of pre-existing conditions or may require a waiting period before coverage for such treatment becomes effective.

- In the context of Medicare, pre-existing conditions are generally not a factor in determining coverage. Original Medicare (consisting of Part A and Part B) does not exclude coverage for treatment of pre-existing conditions, and beneficiaries are not required to undergo a waiting period before receiving coverage for such treatment.

- However, it's important to note that Medicare Advantage plans, which are private health insurance plans that are an alternative to Original Medicare, may have different rules regarding pre-existing conditions. These plans are required to cover everything that Original Medicare covers, but they may have different out-of-pocket costs and may offer additional benefits.

- It's important for beneficiaries to carefully review the terms of their Medicare Advantage plan and understand any potential limitations or exclusions that may apply, including any rules regarding pre-existing conditions.

- Overall, pre-existing conditions are generally not a factor in determining coverage under Original Medicare, but it's important for beneficiaries to understand any potential limitations or exclusions that may apply to Medicare Advantage or Medigap plans.

Premium: The periodic payment to Medicare, an insurance company, or a healthcare plan for health or prescription drug coverage.

- A premium is a periodic payment made to a health insurance plan in exchange for coverage. In the context of Medicare, premiums are paid by beneficiaries for various types of coverage, including Part A (hospital insurance), Part B (medical insurance), and Medicare Advantage or Medigap plans.

- Under Original Medicare (consisting of Part A and Part B), beneficiaries are generally required to pay a premium for Part B coverage. The Part B premium is based on the beneficiary's income and is typically deducted from their Social Security benefit payment.

- For Medicare Part A coverage, most beneficiaries are not required to pay a premium because they or a spouse have paid Medicare taxes while working. However, some beneficiaries may be required to pay a premium if they do not meet the eligibility requirements based on their work history.

- In addition to the Part A and Part B premiums, beneficiaries may also choose to enroll in a Medicare Advantage or Medigap plan, which is a private health insurance plan that is an alternative to Original Medicare. These plans may have different out-of-pocket costs and may offer additional benefits. Premiums for Medicare Advantage plans vary depending on the specific plan chosen.

- Overall, premiums are a periodic payment made by beneficiaries in exchange for coverage under Medicare. It's important for beneficiaries to understand the premiums associated with the various types of coverage available to them and to carefully consider their coverage options.

Preventive Services: Healthcare to prevent illness or detect illness at an early stage, when treatment is likely to work best (for example, preventive services include Pap tests, flu shots, and screening mammograms).

- Preventive services are healthcare services that are provided to help prevent illness or detect medical problems at an early stage when treatment is most likely to be effective. In the context of Medicare, most preventive services are covered under Original Medicare at no cost to the beneficiary.

- Some examples of preventive services covered under Original Medicare include the following:

  - Flu shots

  - Annual wellness visit

  - Bone density test

  - Breast cancer mammogram

  - Colorectal cancer screening

  - Cardiovascular disease screening

  - Diabetes screening

  - Glaucoma tests

  - Prostate cancer screening

- It's important to note that the specific preventive services covered under Original Medicare may vary based on the beneficiary's age, gender, and medical history. It's important for beneficiaries to understand their coverage and to discuss their preventive care needs with their healthcare provider.

- In addition to the preventive services covered under Original Medicare, some Medicare Advantage plans (private health insurance plans that are an alternative to Original Medicare) may also cover additional preventive services. It's important for beneficiaries to understand the terms of their Medicare Advantage plan and to discuss their preventive care needs with their healthcare provider.

- Overall, preventive services are an important tool in maintaining good health and catching potential medical issues early on, and Original Medicare covers a wide range of preventive services at no cost to the beneficiary. It's important for beneficiaries to understand their coverage and to discuss their preventive care needs with their healthcare provider.

Primary Care Doctor: The doctor seen first for most health problems. They make sure an individual gets the care needed to keep the individual healthy. They also may talk with other doctors and healthcare providers about the individual's care and refer the individual to them. In many Medicare Advantage Plans, the beneficiary must see their primary care doctor before they see any other healthcare provider.

- A primary care doctor is a healthcare provider who is responsible for the overall healthcare management of an individual. This may include providing preventive care, diagnosing, and treating medical conditions, and coordinating care with other healthcare providers as needed.

- In the context of Medicare, beneficiaries may choose to see a primary care doctor as part of their Medicare coverage. Under Original Medicare (consisting of Part A and Part B), beneficiaries are generally free to see any healthcare provider who accepts Medicare and who is willing to treat them.

- However, some Medicare Advantage plans (private health insurance plans that are an alternative to Original Medicare) may require beneficiaries to choose a primary care doctor and may require prior authorization before seeing a specialist. It's important for beneficiaries to understand the terms of their Medicare Advantage plan and to discuss their healthcare needs with their primary care doctor.

- Overall, a primary care doctor is an important resource for managing an individual's healthcare and coordinating care with other providers as needed. It's important for Medicare beneficiaries to choose a primary care doctor that they trust and to communicate their healthcare needs and preferences with this provider.

Prior Authorization: Approval that a beneficiary must get from a Medicare drug plan before filling a prescription in order for the prescription to be covered by the plan. The beneficiary's Medicare drug plan may require prior authorization for certain drugs.

- Prior authorization is a process that requires a healthcare provider to obtain approval from a payer (such as Medicare or a private insurance company) before providing certain medical services or prescribing certain medications. The purpose of prior authorization is to ensure that the services or medications are medically necessary and are covered under the individual's insurance plan.

- In the context of Medicare, prior authorization may be required for certain medical services or medications that are considered experimental or not medically necessary. For example, prior authorization may be required for certain outpatient surgeries or for certain medications that are not on the plan's formulary (list of covered drugs).

- Under Original Medicare (consisting of Part A and Part B), prior authorization is generally not required for most medical services and medications. However, some Medicare Advantage plans (private health insurance plans that are an alternative to Original Medicare) may require prior authorization for certain services or medications. It's important for beneficiaries to understand the terms of their Medicare Advantage plan and to discuss any potential prior authorization requirements with their healthcare provider.

- Overall, prior authorization is a process that is used to ensure that medical services and medications are medically necessary and are covered under an individual's insurance plan. It's important for beneficiaries to understand any potential prior authorization requirements and to discuss them with their healthcare provider.

Program of All-Inclusive Care for the Elderly (PACE): A special type of health plan that provides all the care and services covered by Medicare and Medicaid as well as additional medically necessary care and services based on an individual's needs as determined by an interdisciplinary team. PACE serves frail older adults who need nursing home services but are capable of living in the community. PACE combines medical, social, and long-term care services and prescription drug coverage.

- The Program of All-inclusive Care for the Elderly (PACE) is a Medicare and Medicaid program that provides comprehensive medical and social services to seniors who are at risk of nursing home placement. The goal of PACE is to help seniors remain in their homes and communities for as long as possible, while still receiving the care they need.

- To be eligible for PACE, an individual must be fifty-five years of age or older, be certified by the state as needing nursing home level of care and live in a service area that is served by a PACE organization. PACE services are provided through a team of healthcare providers, including doctors, nurses, therapists, and social workers, who work together to develop an individualized care plan for each participant.

- · PACE services may include the following:
- · Primary care
- · Specialty care
- · Inpatient and outpatient hospital care
- · Prescription drugs
- · Home health services
- · Rehabilitation services
- · Social and recreational activities
- · Transportation to and from medical appointments

- PACE is a voluntary program, and beneficiaries may choose to enroll in PACE or to receive their healthcare through other means, such as Original Medicare (consisting of Part A and Part B) or a Medicare Advantage plan. It's important for seniors to consider their healthcare needs and to discuss their options with their healthcare provider.

- Overall, the Program of All-inclusive Care for the Elderly (PACE) is a Medicare and Medicaid program that provides comprehensive medical and social services to seniors who are at risk of nursing home placement. The goal of PACE is to help seniors remain in their homes and communities for as long as possible, while still receiving the care they need.

Q

No Content

R

Referral: A written order from a primary care doctor for a beneficiary to see a specialist or get certain medical services. In many Health Maintenance Organizations (HMOs), a referral is needed before a beneficiary can get medical care from anyone except their primary care doctor. If a referral isn't received first, the plan may not pay for the services.

- A referral is a request from a healthcare provider for an individual to receive medical care from another provider, such as a specialist. In the context of Medicare, referrals may be necessary for beneficiaries to receive certain medical services or to see certain specialists.

- Under Original Medicare (consisting of Part A and Part B), referrals are generally not required for beneficiaries to see specialists. Beneficiaries are generally free to see any healthcare provider who accepts Medicare and who is willing to treat them.

- However, some Medicare Advantage plans (private health insurance plans that are an alternative to Original Medicare) may require beneficiaries to obtain a referral from their primary care doctor before seeing a specialist. It's important for beneficiaries to understand the terms of their Medicare Advantage plan and to discuss any potential referral requirements with their healthcare provider.

- It's also important for beneficiaries to understand that a referral is not the same as a prior authorization, which is a process that requires approval from a payer (such as Medicare or a private insurance company) before providing certain medical services or prescribing certain medications.

- Overall, a referral is a request from a healthcare provider for an individual to receive medical care from another provider. It's important for beneficiaries to understand any potential referral requirements and to discuss them with their healthcare provider.

Rehabilitation Services: Healthcare services that help an individual keep, get back, or improve skills and functioning for daily living that have been lost or if the individual has been impaired because they were sick, hurt, or disabled. These services may include physical and occupational therapy, speech-language pathology, and psychiatric rehabilitation services in a variety of inpatient and/or outpatient settings.

- Rehabilitation services are healthcare services that are designed to help individuals recover from an illness or injury, improve their functioning, and manage their healthcare needs. These services may include physical therapy, occupational therapy, speech-language therapy, and other services to help individuals regain their independence and improve their quality of life.

- In the context of Medicare, rehabilitation services are covered under Original Medicare (consisting of Part A and Part B) when they are medically necessary and are ordered by a healthcare provider. These services may be provided in a variety of settings, including hospitals, skilled nursing facilities, outpatient clinics, and the beneficiary's home.

- Under Original Medicare, beneficiaries are generally required to pay a copayment or coinsurance for rehabilitation services. The amount of the copayment or coinsurance depends on the specific service and the setting in which it is provided.

- In addition to the rehabilitation services covered under Original Medicare, some Medicare Advantage plans (private health insurance plans that are an alternative to Original Medicare) may also cover additional rehabilitation services. It's important for beneficiaries to understand the terms of their Medicare Advantage plan and to discuss their rehabilitation needs with their healthcare provider.

- Overall, rehabilitation services are an important tool in helping individuals recover from an illness or injury and improve their functioning. These services are covered under Original Medicare when they are medically necessary and are ordered by a healthcare provider. It's important for beneficiaries to understand their coverage and to discuss their rehabilitation needs with their healthcare provider.

Religious Nonmedical HealthCare Institution: A facility that provides nonmedical healthcare items and services to people who need hospital or skilled nursing facility care, but for whom that care would be inconsistent with their religious beliefs.

- A religious nonmedical healthcare institution (RNHCI) is a type of healthcare facility that provides nonmedical, supportive care to individuals who are unable to care for themselves due to chronic illness or disability. These facilities are operated by religious organizations and are typically licensed by the state in which they are located.

- In the context of Medicare, RNHCIs may provide certain services that are covered under Original Medicare (consisting of Part A and Part B), such as skilled nursing care and physical therapy. To be eligible for Medicare coverage of these services, the individual must meet certain eligibility requirements, including the following:

- The individual must be receiving services under a plan of care that has been established and periodically reviewed by a doctor.

- The individual must require the services of an SNF or require rehabilitation services on a daily basis.

- The individual must be clinically eligible for the services.

- It's important to note that Medicare does not cover room and board at RNHCIs. However, Medicaid may cover these costs for individuals who meet the income and asset eligibility requirements.

- Overall, an RNHCI is a type of healthcare facility that provides nonmedical, supportive care to individuals who are unable to care for themselves due to chronic illness or disability. These facilities may provide certain services that are covered under Original Medicare, subject to certain eligibility requirements.

Respite Care: Temporary care provided in a nursing home, hospice inpatient facility, or hospital so that a family member or friend who is the patient's caregiver can rest or take some time off.

- Respite care is a type of short-term care that is provided to individuals who need a break from their regular caregiving duties. This type of care is often provided to individuals who are caring for a loved one with a chronic illness or disability, and it is designed to give the caregiver time to rest and recharge.

- In the context of Medicare, respite care is not a covered benefit under Original Medicare (consisting of Part A and Part B). However, respite care may be available through other resources, such as Medicaid or community programs. It's important for caregivers to explore their options and to discuss their needs with their healthcare provider.

- Some Medicare Advantage plans (private health insurance plans that are an alternative to Original Medicare) may offer additional benefits, such as respite care, that are not covered under Original Medicare. It's important for caregivers to understand the terms of their Medicare Advantage plan and to discuss their options with their healthcare provider.

- Overall, respite care is a type of short-term care that is provided to individuals who need a break from their regular caregiving duties. This type of care is not a covered benefit under Original Medicare, but it may be available through other resources. It's important for caregivers to explore their options and to discuss their needs with their healthcare provider.

S

Secondary Payer: The insurance policy, plan, or program that pays second on a claim for medical care. This could be Medicare, Medicaid, or other insurance depending on the situation.

- A secondary payer is a health insurance plan that pays for medical services after another payer, such as Medicare, has made its payment. The secondary payer may be a private insurance plan, such as an employer-sponsored health plan, or it may be a government program, such as Medicaid.

- In the context of Medicare, the secondary payer is responsible for paying any remaining balance after Medicare has made its payment for covered services. The secondary payer may also be responsible for paying for services that are not covered by Medicare.

- It's important for beneficiaries to understand their coverage and to provide their secondary payer information to their healthcare providers so that claims can be properly processed. Beneficiaries should also be aware that they may be responsible for paying any deductibles, copayments, or coinsurance that are not covered by Medicare or the secondary payer.

- Overall, a secondary payer is a health insurance plan that pays for medical services after another payer, such as Medicare, has made its payment. It's important for beneficiaries to understand their coverage and to provide their secondary payer information to their healthcare providers so that claims can be properly processed.

Service Area: A geographic area where the plan accepts members. The plan may limit membership based on where people live. For plans that limit which doctors and hospitals a beneficiary may use, it's also generally the area where a beneficiary can get routine (non-emergency) services. The plan may disenroll the beneficiary if they move out of the plan's service area.

- A service area is the geographic area in which a health insurance plan is available to provide coverage to its beneficiaries. In the context of Medicare, service areas may apply to certain types of coverage, such as Medicare Advantage plans and certain Medicare Part D PDPs.

- Under Original Medicare (consisting of Part A and Part B), beneficiaries are generally free to receive medical care from any healthcare provider who accepts Medicare and who is willing to treat them, regardless of the provider's location.

- However, Medicare Advantage plans (private health insurance plans that are an alternative to Original Medicare) and certain

Medicare Part D PDPs may have service area restrictions. This means that beneficiaries may be required to receive their care from providers within a certain geographic area in order for their care to be covered under the plan.

- It's important for beneficiaries to understand the service area restrictions of their Medicare coverage and to carefully consider their options when choosing a plan. Beneficiaries should also be aware that they may be responsible for paying for care received outside of their plan's service area unless it is an emergency.

- Overall, a service area is the geographic area in which a health insurance plan is available to provide coverage to its beneficiaries. It's important for beneficiaries to understand the service area restrictions of their Medicare coverage and to carefully consider their options when choosing a plan.

Skilled Nursing Care: Care like intravenous injections that can only be given by a registered nurse or doctor.

- Skilled nursing care is a type of medical care that is provided by licensed nurses or other healthcare professionals. This type of care is typically provided to individuals who need a higher level of care than can be provided at home, but who do not need to be hospitalized.

- In the context of Medicare, skilled nursing care is covered under Original Medicare (consisting of Part A and Part B) when it is medically necessary and is ordered by a healthcare provider. To be eligible for Medicare coverage of skilled nursing care, the individual must meet certain eligibility requirements, including the following:

  - The individual must have been hospitalized for at least three consecutive days (not counting the day of discharge).

- The skilled nursing care must be ordered by a doctor.
- The skilled nursing care must be provided by a Medicare-approved facility.
- The skilled nursing care must be medically necessary.

- Under Original Medicare, beneficiaries are generally required to pay a copayment or coinsurance for skilled nursing care. The amount of the copayment or coinsurance depends on the specific service and the setting in which it is provided.

- In addition to the skilled nursing care covered under Original Medicare, some Medicare Advantage plans (private health insurance plans that are an alternative to Original Medicare) may also cover additional skilled nursing care. It's important for beneficiaries to understand the terms of their Medicare Advantage plan and to discuss their skilled nursing care needs with their healthcare provider.

- Overall, skilled nursing care is a type of medical care that is provided by licensed nurses or other healthcare professionals. This type of care is covered under Original Medicare when it is medically necessary and is ordered by a healthcare provider. It's important for beneficiaries to understand their coverage and to discuss their skilled nursing care needs with their healthcare provider.

Skilled Nursing Facility (SNF): A nursing facility with the staff and equipment to give skilled nursing care and, in most cases, skilled rehabilitative services and other related health services.

- An SNF is a type of healthcare facility that provides a higher level of care than can be provided at home, but that is less intensive than inpatient hospital care. SNFs are also known as nursing homes or rehabilitation centers, and they provide a range of services, including skilled nursing care, physical therapy, occupational therapy, and speech-language therapy.

- In the context of Medicare, SNFs are covered under Original Medicare (consisting of Part A and Part B) when they are medically necessary and are ordered by a healthcare provider. To be eligible for Medicare coverage of SNF care, the individual must meet certain eligibility requirements, including the following:

  · The individual must have been hospitalized for at least three consecutive days (not counting the day of discharge).

  · The SNF care must be ordered by a doctor.

  · The SNF care must be provided by a Medicare-approved facility.

  · The SNF care must be medically necessary.

- Under Original Medicare, beneficiaries are generally required to pay a copayment or coinsurance for SNF care. The amount of the copayment or coinsurance depends on the specific service and the length of stay in the SNF.

- In addition to the SNF care covered under Original Medicare, some Medicare Advantage plans (private health insurance plans that are an alternative to Original Medicare) may also cover additional SNF care. It's important for beneficiaries to understand the terms of their Medicare Advantage plan and to discuss their SNF care needs with their healthcare provider.

- Overall, an SNF is a type of healthcare facility that provides a higher level of care than can be provided at home, but that is less intensive than inpatient hospital care. SNFs are covered under Original Medicare when they are medically necessary and are ordered by a healthcare provider. It's important for beneficiaries to understand their coverage and to discuss their SNF care needs with their healthcare provider.

Skilled Nursing Facility (SNF) Care: Skilled nursing care and therapy services provided on a daily basis, in an SNF. Examples of SNF care include physical therapy or intravenous injections that can only be given by a physical therapist or a registered nurse.

- SNF care is a type of medical care that is provided in a healthcare facility, such as a nursing home or rehabilitation center. SNF care is typically provided to individuals who need a higher level of care than can be provided at home, but who do not need to be hospitalized. This type of care may include skilled nursing care, physical therapy, occupational therapy, and speech-language therapy.

- SNF care is typically provided by a team of healthcare professionals, including doctors, nurses, therapists, and social workers. The team works together to develop an individualized care plan for each patient, with the goal of helping the patient regain their independence and improve their quality of life.

- SNF care is generally necessary for individuals who are unable to perform daily activities, such as bathing, dressing, and using the bathroom, on their own. It may also be necessary for individuals who require ongoing medical supervision or who need rehabilitation services to recover from an illness or injury.

- SNF care is typically covered by health insurance, including Medicare and Medicaid. It's important for individuals to understand their coverage and to discuss their SNF care needs with their healthcare provider.

- Overall, SNF care is a type of medical care that is provided in a healthcare facility to individuals who need a higher level of care than can be provided at home, but who do not need to be hospitalized. This type of care is typically covered by health insurance and is provided by a team of healthcare professionals who work together to develop an individualized care plan.

Special Enrollment Period (SEP): You can make changes to your Medicare Advantage and Medicare prescription drug coverage when certain events happen in your life, like if you move or you lose other insurance coverage. These chances to make changes are called Special Enrollment Periods (SEPs). Rules about when you can make changes and the type of changes you can make are different for each SEP.

State Health Insurance Assistance Program (SHIP): A state program that gets money from the federal government to give free local health insurance counseling to people with Medicare.

- The SHIP is a free, unbiased counseling service that is provided by the U.S. Government to help individuals with Medicare understand their options and make informed decisions about their healthcare coverage. SHIP is funded through the CMS and is administered by the states.

- SHIP counselors are trained to provide personalized assistance to individuals with Medicare and their families. They can help beneficiaries understand their Medicare coverage options, including Original Medicare (consisting of Part A and Part B), Medicare Advantage plans, and Medicare Part D PDPs. They can also provide information on Medicare supplements (also known as Medigap policies), which can help cover out-of-pocket costs under Original Medicare.

- SHIP counselors can also provide assistance with enrolling in Medicare, filing appeals, and understanding Medicare billing and claims. They can provide assistance in person, over the phone, or online, depending on the state in which the individual resides.

- SHIP counselors are trained to provide personalized assistance to individuals with Medicare and their families.

State Insurance Department: A state agency that regulates insurance and can provide information about Medigap policies and other private health insurance.

- The state insurance department is a government agency that is responsible for regulating the insurance industry within a state. In the context of Medigap policies and other private health insurance, the state insurance department can provide information and assistance to individuals who have questions about their coverage.

- Medigap policies are private health insurance policies that are designed to supplement Original Medicare (consisting of Part A and Part B). They can help cover out-of-pocket costs, such as deductibles, copayments, and coinsurance, that are not covered under Original Medicare. Medigap policies are standardized by the federal government, but they are sold by private insurance companies.

- Individuals with Medigap policies or other private health insurance can contact their state insurance department for assistance with a variety of issues, including the following:

  - Understanding their policy benefits and coverage limits
  - Enrolling in a Medigap policy or making changes to their coverage

- Filing appeals or resolving disputes with their insurance plan
- Understanding billing and claims processes
- Finding financial assistance for premiums, deductibles, and copayments

- The state insurance department can also provide information on other types of health insurance coverage that may be available in the state, such as Medicare Advantage plans or employer-sponsored health plans.

State Medical Assistance (Medicaid) Office: A state or local agency that can give information about, and help with applications for, Medicaid programs that help pay medical bills for people with limited income and resources.

- State Medical Assistance, also known as Medicaid, is a joint federal and state program that provides health insurance coverage to low-income individuals and families. Medicaid is administered by the states, and each state has its own Medicaid program with its own eligibility requirements and covered benefits.

- In general, Medicaid is available to people with low incomes, including children, pregnant women, parents, seniors, and people with disabilities. Medicaid also covers certain low-income adults without children. To be eligible for Medicaid, an individual must meet certain income and asset limits, which vary by state.

- Medicaid is an important source of health coverage for many Americans. According to the CMS, as of 2020, more than 75 million people were enrolled in Medicaid, including nearly 40 million children. Medicaid provides a wide range of benefits, including physician and hospital services, prescription drugs, and long-term care services such as nursing home care.

- The State Medical Assistance office is responsible for administering the Medicaid program in each state. This includes determining eligibility for Medicaid, enrolling eligible individuals in the program, and paying claims for covered benefits. The State Medical Assistance office may also be responsible for coordinating with other state agencies and organizations to ensure that Medicaid beneficiaries have access to the care and services they need.

- If an individual is interested in applying for Medicaid, they can contact their state's Medicaid office for more information. An individual can also visit the CMS website, which has a list of state Medicaid programs and links to their websites. Additionally, an individual may be able to apply for Medicaid online through their state's healthcare exchange or through the federal healthcare marketplace.

- Overall, the State Medical Assistance office plays a crucial role in providing health insurance coverage to low-income individuals and families through the Medicaid program. If an individual may be eligible for Medicaid, it is important to explore all options and apply for coverage if needed.

State Pharmaceutical Assistance Program (SPAP): A state program that provides help paying for drug coverage based on financial need, age, or medical condition.

- State Pharmaceutical Assistance Programs (SPAPs) are state-funded programs that help low-income individuals pay for their prescription medications. SPAPs are designed to assist seniors and people with disabilities who have high out-of-pocket costs for their medications, but who do not qualify for Medicaid or other federal assistance programs.

- Each state has its own SPAP, and the eligibility requirements and covered medications vary by state. To be eligible for an SPAP, an individual must meet certain income and asset limits and may also need to be enrolled in Medicare Part D, a federal program that provides prescription drug coverage.

- SPAPs may provide financial assistance for all or some of the medications on an individual's PDP. Some SPAPs also have a list of medications that they cover, which may be different from the list of medications covered by an individual's Medicare Part D plan.

- To apply for an SPAP, beneficiaries can contact their state's SPAP office or visit the website of their state's SPAP. Beneficiaries may need to provide information about their income, assets, and medications, and they may also need to provide proof of their Medicare Part D enrollment.

- Overall, SPAPs are an important resource for low-income individuals who have high out-of-pocket costs for their prescription medications. If a beneficiary may be eligible for an SPAP, it is important to explore all options and apply for assistance if needed.

State Survey Agency: A state agency that oversees healthcare facilities that participate in the Medicare and/or Medicaid programs by, for example, inspecting healthcare facilities and investigating complaints to ensure that health and safety standards are met.

- State Survey Agencies are responsible for ensuring that healt-care facilities, including hospitals, nursing homes, and home health agencies, meet state and federal regulations and standards. State

Survey Agencies are typically part of the state's Department of Health and are responsible for conducting surveys, inspections, and complaint investigations at healthcare facilities.

- The primary goal of State Survey Agencies is to protect the health and safety of patients and residents in healthcare facilities. To do this, they conduct surveys and inspections to ensure that facilities are in compliance with regulations and standards related to patient care, quality of life, and facility operations. This may include checking for issues such as inadequate staffing levels, inadequate infection control measures, and failure to follow appropriate care protocols.

- State Survey Agencies also investigate complaints about healthcare facilities. If a patient, resident, or family member has a concern or complaint about the care or treatment received at a healthcare facility, they can contact the State Survey Agency to file a report. The State Survey Agency will then investigate the complaint and take appropriate action if necessary.

- If a healthcare facility is found to be out of compliance with regulations or standards, the State Survey Agency may take a variety of corrective actions, such as requiring the facility to make changes or improvements, issuing fines, or revoking the facility's license.

- Overall, the State Survey Agency plays a critical role in ensuring the quality and safety of care in healthcare facilities. If beneficiaries have concerns or complaints about a healthcare facility, they can contact their state's State Survey Agency for assistance.

Step Therapy: A coverage rule used by some Medicare Prescription Drug Plans that requires a beneficiary to try one or more similar, lower cost drugs to treat their condition before the plan will cover the prescribed drug.

- Step therapy, also known as "fail first" or "sequential therapy," is a cost-control measure used by insurance companies and pharmacy benefit managers (PBMs) to encourage the use of less expensive medications before more expensive ones. With step therapy, an individual with a prescription for a certain medication must first try a less expensive medication (or a set of medications) before the insurance plan will cover the cost of the originally prescribed medication.

- Step therapy is often used for medications that are used to treat chronic conditions, such as diabetes, high blood pressure, and mental health disorders. The goal of step therapy is to ensure that individuals are using the most cost-effective medications available, but it can also be used to encourage the use of generic medications over brand-name medications.

- Step therapy can be frustrating for individuals and their healthcare providers, as it can delay access to the most appropriate treatment. For example, if an individual has tried a less expensive medication in the past and it was not effective, they may have to try multiple other medications before they can get coverage for the medication that their healthcare provider originally prescribed.

- There are some exceptions to step therapy, such as in the case of an allergic reaction or other contraindication to a specific medication. Additionally, some states have laws that limit the use of step therapy or require insurance plans to have an "exception process" in place for individuals who are unable to use the required medications due to medical necessity.

- Overall, step therapy is a cost-control measure that is used by insurance plans and PBMs to encourage the use of less expensive medications. While it can be frustrating for individuals and their healthcare providers, it is important to work with the insurance plan and the healthcare provider to ensure that the individual is receiving the most appropriate and effective treatment for their condition.

Supplemental Security Income (SSI): A monthly benefit paid by Social Security to people with limited income and resources who are disabled, blind, or age sixty-five or older. SSI benefits aren't the same as Social Security retirement or disability benefits.

- SSI is a federal program that provides financial assistance to low-income individuals who are aged sixty-five or older, blind, or disabled. SSI is designed to help individuals meet their basic needs, such as food, clothing, and shelter.

- To be eligible for SSI, an individual must meet certain income and asset limits. Income includes wages, self-employment income, and any other money that an individual receives, such as Social Security benefits or pensions. Assets include things like cash, savings accounts, stocks, and property (excluding the individual's primary residence).

- The amount of SSI that an individual receives is based on their income and assets, as well as the cost of living in the area where they live. SSI payments are generally made on a monthly basis and are adjusted for inflation each year.

- In addition to financial assistance, SSI also provides individuals with automatic eligibility for Medicaid, a federal and state program that provides health insurance coverage to low-income individuals.

- To apply for SSI, individuals can visit the SSA website or visit a local SSA office. The application process may include completing an application form, providing proof of income and assets, and providing proof of age, blindness, or disability.

- Overall, SSI is an important program that provides financial assistance to low-income individuals who are aged sixty-five or older, blind, or disabled. If an individual may be eligible for SSI, it is important to explore all options and apply for assistance if needed.

Supplier: Generally, any company, person, or agency that supplies a medical item or service, except when an individual is an inpatient in a hospital or skilled nursing facility.

- A supplier is a business or individual that provides DME, prosthetics, orthotics, and other medical supplies to Medicare beneficiaries. Medicare-approved suppliers must meet certain requirements in order to be able to bill Medicare for the items and services they provide.

- DME is equipment that is used in the home and is primarily used to serve a medical purpose. Examples of DME include hospital beds, wheelchairs, oxygen equipment, and blood sugar monitors. Medicare covers the cost of DME if it is medically necessary and ordered by a healthcare provider.

- Prosthetics are artificial limbs or devices that are used to replace a missing body part or to support a weak or deformed body part. Orthotics are devices that are used to support or correct the function of the body's musculoskeletal system. Medicare covers the cost of prosthetics and orthotics if they are medically necessary and ordered by a healthcare provider.

- To be a Medicare-approved supplier, a business or individual must be enrolled in the Medicare program and meet certain standards. These standards may include having a valid business license, being in compliance with state and local regulations, and having a physical location where the items and services are provided.

- If a Medicare beneficiary needs DME, prosthetics, or orthotics, they should work with a Medicare-approved supplier. Beneficiaries can find a list of Medicare-approved suppliers on the Medicare website or by contacting their local Medicare office.

- Overall, Medicare-approved suppliers are an important resource for Medicare beneficiaries who need DME, prosthetics, and orthotics. It is important to work with a Medicare-approved supplier to ensure that beneficiaries are receiving high-quality items and services that are covered by Medicare.

T

Telemedicine: Medical or other health services given to a patient using a communications system (like a computer, phone, or television) by a practitioner in a location different than the patient's.

- Telemedicine is the use of technology, such as videoconferencing, phone, or email, to provide medical care and services remotely. Telemedicine allows individuals to receive medical care from the comfort of their own home or other location, rather than having to travel to a healthcare facility.

- Medicare, the federal health insurance program for individuals who are aged sixty-five or older or who have certain disabilities, covers certain telemedicine services. Medicare coverage of telemedicine varies depending on the type of service and the location of the beneficiary.

- In general, Medicare covers telemedicine services that are provided by a healthcare professional and that are medically necessary. This may include services such as virtual check-ins, e-visits, and remote monitoring. Medicare may also cover telemedicine services that are provided as part of a clinical trial or as a follow-up to an in-person visit.

- To be eligible for Medicare coverage of telemedicine services, an individual must be located in a rural area or in an area that is designated as a Health Professional Shortage Area. Additionally, the individual must be receiving the telemedicine services from a healthcare professional who is enrolled in the Medicare program and who is authorized to provide the service in the state where the individual is located.

- If a Medicare beneficiary is interested in receiving telemedicine services, they should check with their healthcare provider to see if telemedicine services are offered and to verify if those services are covered by Medicare. Beneficiaries can also visit the Medicare website to learn more about coverage of telemedicine services.

- Overall, telemedicine is an important tool that allows individuals to receive medical care remotely, and Medicare covers certain telemedicine services for eligible beneficiaries. If a Medicare beneficiary is interested in receiving telemedicine services, it is important to check with their healthcare provider and their Medicare plan to see what is covered.

Tiers: Groups of drugs that have a different cost for each group. Generally, a drug in a lower tier will cost less than a drug in a higher tier.

- Tiers refer to the levels of cost-sharing that apply to medications. PDPs, including those offered by private insurance companies and Medicare Part D, divide medications into different tiers, with each tier having a different level of cost-sharing.

- The number of tiers and the specific medications that are included in each tier can vary depending on the plan. In general, the higher the tier, the higher the cost-sharing for the medications in that tier.

- The most common tiers are:

  · Tier 1: Generic medications. These are medications that have the same active ingredients as a brand-name medication, but they are generally less expensive.

  · Tier 2: Preferred brand-name medications. These are brand-name medications that have been approved by the plan and that have been found to be safe and effective.

  · Tier 3: Nonpreferred brand-name medications. These are brand-name medications that are not on the preferred list and that may not have been found to be as safe and effective as medications on the preferred list.

  · Tier 4: Specialty medications. These are medications that are used to treat complex or rare conditions and that may be very expensive.

- The cost-sharing for each tier can vary depending on the plan. Some plans may have a copayment (a fixed amount that the individual pays each time they fill a prescription) for each tier, while others may have a coinsurance (a percentage of the cost of the medication that the individual pays).

- It is important for individuals to understand the tiers and the cost-sharing for their PDP, as this can help them make informed decisions about their medications. If beneficiaries have questions about the tiers and cost-sharing for their plan, they should contact their plan or visit their website for more information.

TTY: A TTY (teletypewriter) is a communication device used by people who are deaf, hard-of-hearing, or have severe speech impairment. People who don't have a TTY can communicate with a TTY user through a message relay center (MRC). An MRC has TTY operators available to send and interpret TTY messages.

- A TTY (teletypewriter) is a device that allows individuals who are deaf, hard of hearing, or speech-impaired to communicate over the phone using text. TTYs are also known as TDDs (telecommunications display devices) or text telephones.

- In the context of Medicare, a TTY is a device that is covered under Medicare Part B (Medical Insurance) if it is medically necessary and prescribed by a healthcare provider. Medicare Part B covers the rental or purchase of TTYs for individuals who are deaf, hard of hearing, or speech-impaired and who have difficulty using the phone because of their disability.

- To be eligible for coverage of a TTY under Medicare Part B, an individual must have a written prescription from a healthcare provider. The individual must also meet certain eligibility requirements, such as being enrolled in Medicare Part B and being a resident of the United States.

- If a Medicare beneficiary is deaf, hard of hearing, or speech-impaired and they have difficulty using the phone because of the disability, they may be eligible for coverage of a TTY under Medicare Part B. Beneficiaries should contact their healthcare provider to discuss the options and to get a written prescription for a TTY. Beneficiaries can also contact their local Medicare office or visit the Medicare website for more information.

- Overall, TTYs are an important tool that allows individuals who are deaf, hard of hearing, or speech-impaired to communicate over the phone using text. If a Medicare beneficiary may be eligible for coverage of a TTY, it is important to explore all options and to work with a healthcare provider to get the device that is right.

U

Urgently needed care: Care that a beneficiary receives outside of their Medicare health plan's service area for a sudden illness or injury that needs medical care right away but isn't life threatening. If it's not safe to wait until a beneficiary arrives home to get care from a plan doctor, the health plan must pay for the care.

- Urgently needed care refers to medical care that is needed right away because of an illness, injury, or other health condition that cannot wait until the individual's next scheduled appointment. Urgently needed care may be needed outside of normal office hours or on holidays, and it may include services such as emergency department visits, urgent care visits, or home visits.

- In the context of Medicare, urgently needed care is covered under Medicare Part B (Medical Insurance) if it is medically necessary and provided by a Medicare-approved provider. Medicare Part B covers a wide range of medical services, including emergency department visits, urgent care visits, and home visits.

- To receive coverage for urgently needed care under Medicare Part B, an individual must be enrolled in Medicare Part B and must meet certain eligibility requirements. The individual must also see a Medicare-approved provider and must receive services that are medically necessary.

- If a Medicare beneficiary needs urgently needed care, it is important they contact their healthcare provider or seek care at a Medicare-approved facility, such as an emergency department or urgent care center. If a beneficiary is unsure about where to go for urgently needed care, they can call a local Medicare office or the Medicare hotline for assistance.

- Overall, urgently needed care is an important component of the Medicare program, as it ensures that individuals can receive the medical care they need in a timely manner, even outside of normal office hours or on holidays. If a Medicare beneficiary needs urgently needed care, it is important to seek care from a Medicare-approved provider to ensure that their care is covered by Medicare.

V

No Content

W

Workers' compensation: An insurance plan that employers are required to have to cover employees who get sick or injured on the job.

- Workers' compensation is a type of insurance that covers medical expenses and lost wages for individuals who are injured on the job. Workers' compensation is provided by the employer and is typically required by state law.

- In the context of Medicare, workers' compensation is a secondary payer to Medicare. This means that if an individual receives workers' compensation benefits for a work-related injury or illness, Medicare may pay for some of the medical expenses that are not covered by workers' compensation.

- If an individual is receiving workers' compensation benefits, Medicare may pay for medical expenses that are not covered by workers' compensation if the expenses are medically necessary and reasonable. Medicare may also pay for medical expenses that are related to a work-related injury or illness, even if the individual is not receiving workers' compensation benefits.

- It is important for individuals who are receiving workers' compensation benefits to notify their workers' compensation insurer and their Medicare plan about the injury or illness, as this can help ensure that their medical expenses are covered by the appropriate payer.

- If a Medicare beneficiary is receiving workers' compensation benefits for a work-related injury or illness, it is important to notify the workers' compensation insurer and the Medicare plan about the injury or illness. The beneficiary should also keep track of their medical expenses and receipts, as you may need to provide.

X

No Content

Y

No Content

Z

No Content

NOTES

NOTES

NOTES

NOTES

NOTES

NOTES